Rheumatology
of the Upper Limbs
in Clinical Practice

José António Pereira da Silva
Anthony D. Woolf

Rheumatology of the Upper Limbs in Clinical Practice

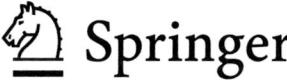 Springer

Dr. José António Pereira da Silva
MD. PhD
Department of Rheumatology
University Hospital
Coimbra
Portugal

Dr. Anthony D. Woolf, MSc, MBBS
FRCP
Department of Rheumatology
Royal Cornwall Hospital
Truro
United Kingdom

First published in 2010 as part of Rheumatology in Practice
(ISBN 978-1-84882-580-2)

Rheumatology in Practice (ISBN 978-1-84882-580-2) was previously
published in Portuguese by **Diagnósteo** as *Reumatologia Prática* by
José António Pereira da Silva, 2005.

ISBN 978-1-4471-2241-8   e-ISBN 978-1-4471-2242-5
DOI 10.1007/978-1-4471-2242-5
Springer London Dordrecht Heidelberg New York

British Library Cataloguing in Publication Data
A catalogue record for this book is available from the British Library

Library of Congress Control Number: 2011944216

Printed on acid-free paper

Springer is part of Springer Science+Business Media (www.springer.com)

Contents

GUIDE

TYPICAL CASES

MAIN POINTS

UNDERLINED

TABLES

Chapter 1
Regional Syndromes
The Painful Shoulder

Pain in the shoulder region is a common reason for seeking medical attention. When shoulder pain presents as an isolated problem, the cause is usually periarticular disease that can be diagnosed accurately by clinical examination. It is not uncommon for shoulder pain to be referred from adjacent areas or internal organs. While isolated affection of the glenohumeral joint is rare, this joint is often involved in a variety of polyarthropathies.

Shoulder pain is often extremely incapacitating. Conservative treatment is usually highly satisfactory.

Functional Anatomy

The shoulder is an extremely complex structure.

Take a moment to imagine a mechanical structure capable of carrying out all the shoulder's movements: adduction, abduction, flexion (anterior elevation) and extension in an arc greater than 180°. The hand can reach any point within more than half a circle with a radius similar to the length of the upper limb! In addition, this mechanical structure should be able to rotate round its own axis – internal and external rotation – and to provide considerable force. This mobility requires considerable strength from the soft supporting structures, which results in considerable risk of instability. If we add

J.A.P. da Silva, A.D. Woolf, *Rheumatology of the Upper Limbs in Clinical Practice*, DOI 10.1007/978-1-4471-2242-5_1, © Springer-Verlag London Limited 2012

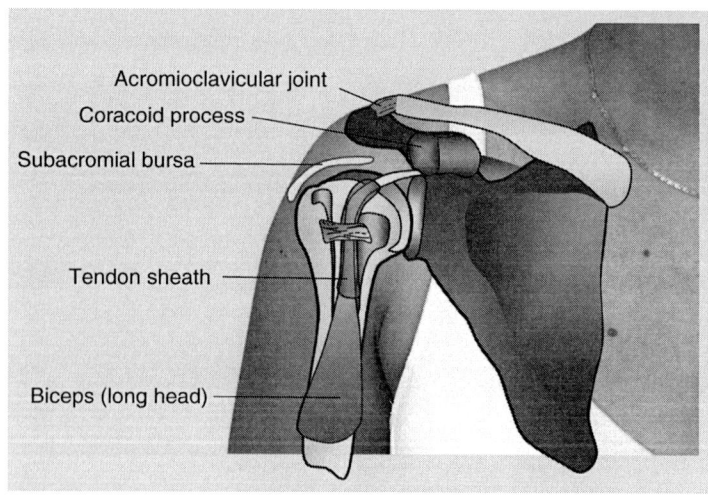

Acromioclavicular joint

Coracoid process

Subacromial bursa

Tendon sheath

Biceps (long head)

FIGURE 1.1 Functional anatomy of the shoulder

all this to the need for a control system capable of conducting all these movements smoothly and accurately, we are looking at an amazing structure! There is no way it could be simple.

The shoulder consists of three bones and three joints. The proximal end of the humerus, the scapula and the lateral end of the clavicle come together here (Fig. 1.1).

The humerus articulates with the glenoid surface of the scapula, amplified by a cartilaginous ring (the glenoid labrum), making the glenohumeral joint, which has a synovial lining and is strengthened by a fibrous capsule and ligaments. It is the most mobile joint in the whole body and is involved in rotation, flexion, extension, and a substantial amount of adduction and abduction (between 0 and 120°).

Above the glenohumeral joint is the acromioclavicular joint, which joins the lateral end of the clavicle to the internal edge of the acromion. Anteriorly, the coracoacromial ligament continues coverage of the head of the humerus and adjacent structures.

The scapula glides over the subscapularis muscle and the muscles of the posterior thoracic wall, suspended by muscles responsible for elevation and internal and external rotation: the elevator muscle of the scapula, serratus anterior, trapezium and rhomboids, among others. It thus constitutes what we call the scapulothoracic joint, which plays an important part in all the movements of the shoulder: abduction between 120 and 180°, and part of extension, and internal and external rotation.

The shoulder is served by a complex set of muscles. Externally, the deltoid arises from the lateral third of the clavicle, the border of the acromion and along the spine of the scapula. Below, it inserts into the lateral aspect of the humerus. It is divided into three parts: anterior, external and posterior, which induce flexion, abduction and extension, respectively. It is responsible for abduction of the arm between 30 and 90°. Over 90°, abduction is the result of the contraction of trapezius, which elevates the scapula and clavicle.

The first 30° of abduction depend on the contraction of the supraspinatus. This muscle is part of the so-called rotator cuff of the shoulder. This is the name given to the musculotendinous structure that results from the junction of the tendons of four muscles joining the scapula to the humerus: the supraspinatus, infraspinatus, subscapularis and teres minor. The tendons of the muscles in the rotator cuff are inserted externally along the anatomical neck of the humerus (Figs. 1.2 and 1.3). The supraspinatus tendon inserts in the greater tuberosity of the humerus, a bony prominence lateral to the head of the humerus. The infraspinatus inserts posteriorly and induces external rotation with the support of the teres minor, with slightly more distal insertion in the posterior aspect. The subscapularis inserts in the lesser tuberosity of the humerus along the internal border of the bicipital groove of the humerus. Its contraction induces internal rotation of the shoulder.

Anteriorly, the predominant muscle is biceps brachialis. It inserts inferiorly via a common tendon in the radial tuberosity. The upper part of the biceps is divided in two. The inner part, the short head of the biceps, inserts in the coracoid process of the scapula. The long head of biceps becomes a long tendon that runs on the anterior aspect of the humerus (the intertubercular sulcus or bicipital groove) and through the

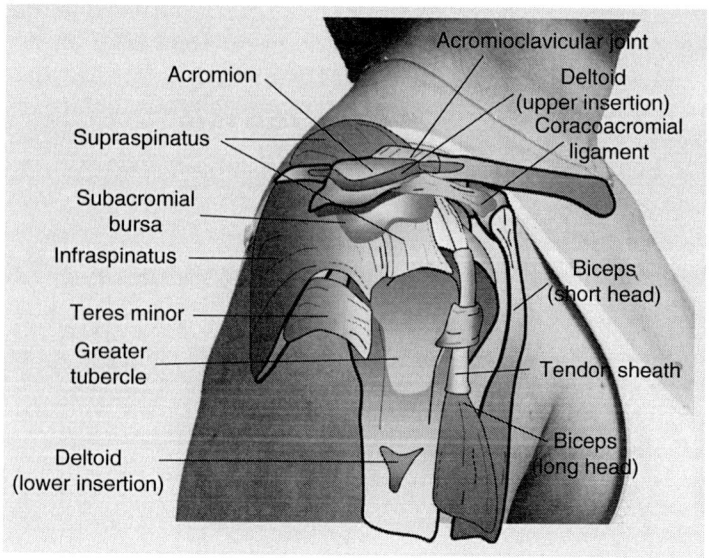

FIGURE 1.2 The rotator cuff of the shoulder and its anatomical relations

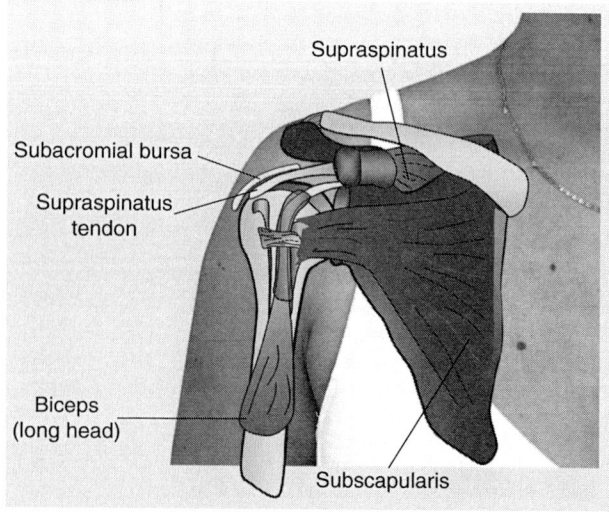

FIGURE 1.3 Functional anatomy of the shoulder. Internal rotation

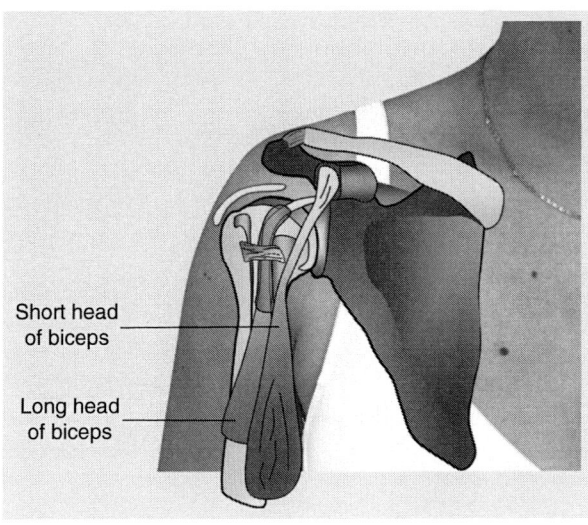

Short head
of biceps

Long head
of biceps

FIGURE 1.4 Functional anatomy of the shoulder. Short and long head of biceps

glenohumeral joint to insert in the upper aspect of the glenoid cavity of the scapula. This tendon is coated with a long synovial sheath along the upper third of the humerus, which is a common site of inflammation (Fig. 1.4).

Contraction of the biceps naturally induces flexion of the humerus at the shoulder and flexion of the forearm on the upper arm. Given that the radial tuberosity is located in the medial aspect the radius, the biceps promotes the supination of the hand and forearm.

Other muscles are involved in the movements of the shoulder: the pectoralis major and latissimus dorsi, which are responsible for adduction, and the teres major. The triceps and rhomboid support the swinging movements of the scapula.

The upper outer quadrant of the shoulder is a problem area, with frequent conflicts of space. Above, the acromion forms a rigid, unyielding ceiling. Below, is the supraspinatus tendon, which pulls the head of the humerus upwards every time it contracts, reducing an already limited space.

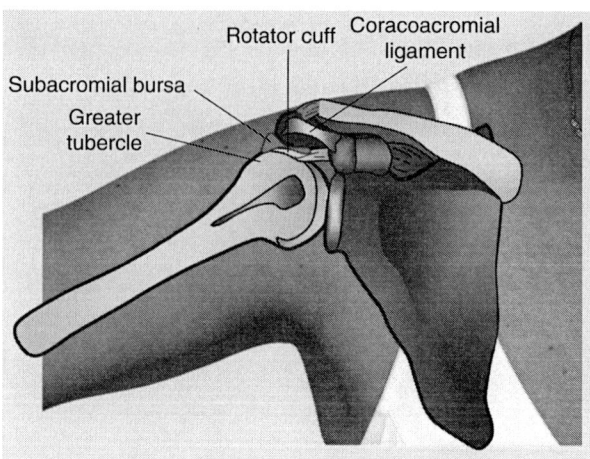

FIGURE 1.5 Subacromial impingement

In addition, complete abduction means that the greater tuberosity enters the space.[1]

There is a synovial bursa that helps these structures to glide more easily: the subacromial bursa. Understandably, this structure, together with the rotator cuff, is exposed to the repeated friction trauma that may result in painful, incapacitating local inflammation (Fig. 1.5).

Radiological Anatomy

An anteroposterior x-ray of the shoulder in a neutral position (Fig. 1.6) enables us to assess the regularity of the

---

[1]Try elevating your arms in abduction up to 180°, keeping the palms of your hands facing down. Did you manage? Congratulations! Many people cannot do it without rotating their palms upwards when they reach about 90° abduction because there is not enough subacromial space to accommodate the greater tuberosity. They are therefore forced to induce external rotation of the humerus, moving the greater tuberosity behind the acromion.

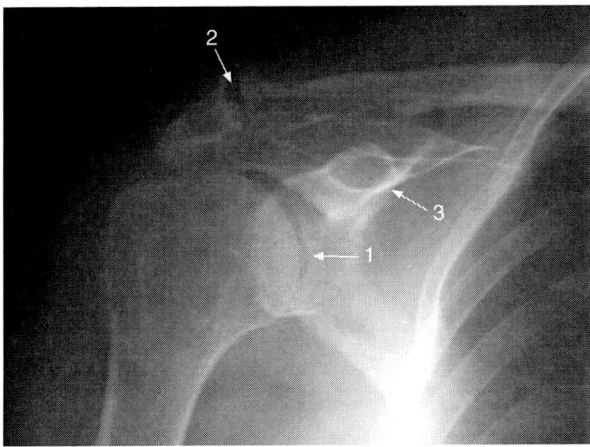

FIGURE 1.6 Normal radiology of the shoulder (right shoulder in neutral position). *1* Gleno-humeral joint. *2* Acromio-clavicular joint. *3* Coracoid process of the scapula

glenoid cavity of the scapula, the head of the humerus and the greater tuberosity and any calcification of the rotator cuff or subacromial bursa. Acromioclavicular osteoarthritis may require a special view. The distance between the lowest point of the acromioclavicular joint and the highest point of the head of the humerus should be at least 5 mm. Any less suggests a rupture of the supraspinatus tendon. The view in internal rotation (Fig. 1.7) makes it possible to assess the rest of the head of the humerus: sphericity, regularity, and the subchondral bone. In both views, look for possible lytic or sclerotic lesions.

Common Causes of Shoulder Pain

Until proven otherwise, isolated pain in the shoulder is likely to be of periarticular origin. Periarticular lesions of the shoulder are extremely common, while isolated disease of the glenohumeral joint is rare.

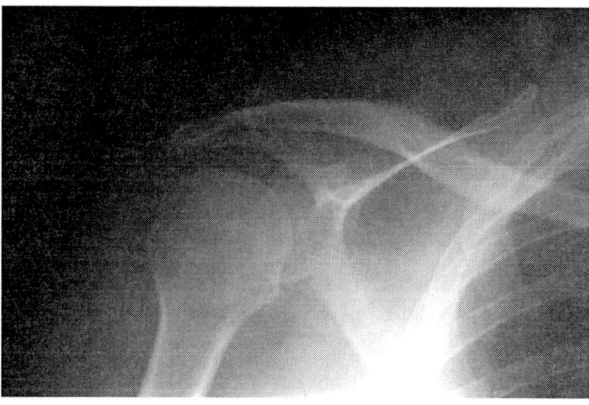

FIGURE 1.7 Normal radiology of the shoulder (AP view of the right shoulder in internal rotation)

Disease of the shoulder is most common in people whose occupation or leisure activities involve repeated movements with the arms raised: cleaners, teachers, agricultural workers, factory workers, professional swimmers etc.

Provided that they are thorough, the enquiry and clinical examination are extremely rewarding, as, in most cases, they allow an accurate diagnosis without the need for diagnostic tests. On the other hand, most of these lesions, which are highly incapacitating, can be treated effectively with simple techniques, which is very rewarding both for the patient and the doctor.

Table 1.1 shows the most common causes of shoulder pain.

The Enquiry

The first aim of the enquiry is to find out whether the problem is limited to the shoulder or is part of a more widespread disease. Knowing the patient's occupational and leisure activities and assessing any chronic concomitant diseases such as diabetes mellitus, sequelae of a cerebrovascular accident, previous heart surgery or myocardial infarction, etc. can give us important clues. A history of trauma or a fall is particularly relevant.

TABLE 1.1 Common causes of shoulder pain

Etiology	Clinical clues
Tendonitis of the supraspinatus or infraspinatus and subacromial bursitis	Localized pain in the shoulder or upper arm Worse during abduction Nocturnal pain common – unable to sleep on same side Specific maneuvers in the clinical examination
Tendonitis of the long head of the biceps	Pain mainly in the anterior aspect of the shoulder Worse during flexion Specific maneuvers in the clinical examination
Adhesive capsulitis ("Frozen shoulder")	Diffuse shoulder pain Limitation of all movements during active and passive mobilization*
Complete tear (rupture) of the supraspinatus	Pain similar to tendonitis of the supraspinatus Complete active abduction impossible
Referred pain	Diffuse Unrelated to movements of the shoulder Normal local and regional clinical examination
Glenohumeral arthritis	Inflammatory pain Pain on active and passive mobilization Limited active and passive mobility More joints usually involved
Acromioclavicular disease and instability	Pain in the upper aspect of the shoulder Mechanical pain Worse during extreme abduction
Glenohumeral instability	Most common in young people Recurring

NB: capsulitis has clinical characteristics suggesting joint disease

The onset of periarticular lesions tends to be sudden or subacute, quite often related to a precise moment or gesture. Rupture of the supraspinatus is usually preceded by prolonged suffering with repeated episodes of pain.

Selectivity of painful movements is highly suggestive of a periarticular lesion and even of its type. Is the pain worse with movement? Is there a particularly painful movement? Abduction? Flexion? Patients with a periarticular lesion often say that the pain is worse at night, especially when lying on the same side. This is common to arthritis however and is not much use to differential diagnosis.

If the pain does not get worse during movement of the shoulder, we should look for causes of referred pain. Neurogenic radiated pain (of cervical origin) is suggested by dysesthesia and concomitant neck pain radiating to the shoulder and/or upper limb. As a rule, in these cases, movement of the neck exacerbates the pain in the shoulder. Questions about coronary, respiratory and biliary problems are mandatory.

If the pain also affects other articular areas, we must ascertain their nature, exploring the possibility polyarthropathy with shoulder involvement. We should not, however, ignore the fact that the association of periarticular lesions, of the shoulder and hand, for example, is quite common and can be misleading. Shoulder pain is also common in patients with fibromyalgia, but there is usually generalized pain, which is suggestive of this diagnosis.

Regional Examination

Observation

Surface observation of the shoulder is relatively unproductive, as the glenohumeral joint is deep-set and protected by muscle. Only rarely are intra-articular effusions or effusions from the bursae visible as an area of fullness on the anterior face of the shoulder. For the same reason, redness is unusual, even in cases of intense synovitis. Swelling of the acromio-clavicular joint is easily visible and palpable.

Rupture of the supraspinatus tendon, severe lesions of the cervical roots or the brachial plexus and prolonged disuse can cause atrophy of the shoulder muscles, which is easy to see when it involves the supraspinatus or infraspinatus.

Mobilization

This is the fundamental part of a clinical examination of the shoulder and should involve three different aspects:

a. *Active mobilization* – the patient carries out the movement unaided.
b. *Passive mobilization* – the examiner carries out the movement while the patient remains as relaxed as possible.
c. *Resisted mobilization* – the patient is asked to carry out the movement while the examiner offers resistance.

If active mobilization is free, full-range and painless, it is unlikely to be any significant pathology of the shoulder, as all the articular and periarticular structures take part in the movement.

If active mobilization is painful or limited in range, assessment of passive mobilization should follow. When the patient is relaxed, passive mobilization involves the joints and capsules, but leaves the tendons at rest. If passive mobilization is much less painful or less limited in range than active mobilization, the problem is much more likely to be periarticular and not articular. The opposite is the case if the pain and range restriction are similar during active and passive mobilization.

Resisted mobilization places tendons and bursae under tension, which causes intense pain if these structures have lesions. The appropriate maneuvers are well defined so that each one assesses specific structures. They must be carried out properly because if not interpretation will be erroneous.

Main Points

In periarticular lesions, there is pain in selected active and resisted movements. Movement range can be reduced by pain. Passive mobilization is more ample and less painful than active mobilization.

In adhesive capsulitis and diseases of the glenohumeral joint, all active and passive movements are painful and frequently limited in range. The range of passive movements is also reduced. Resisted movements cause little or no exacerbation of pain.

The shoulder is already assessed to a reasonable extent in the general examination. If the patient complains of shoulder pain, either spontaneously or during the examination, or if mobility is significantly limited, a more detailed examination is necessary.

The method we suggest is as follows:

a. The patient is asked to repeat total abduction of the arm to 180°, if possible, telling us as soon as he feels pain and whether it goes away as he continues the movement. We suggest that you show the patient the movement and ask him to repeat it.

Normally, in supraspinatus tendonitis or subacromial bursitis, this maneuver causes pain in an arc between 30 and 120°, subsiding above this angle. In more severe cases, the pain may force the patient to interrupt the movement. If the patient is unable to maintain his shoulder at 90° after passive abduction, a rupture of the supraspinatus is highly probable. Pain that only appears above 120° abduction suggests osteoarthritis of the acromioclavicular joint (Fig. 1.8).

b. We then ask the patient to raise his arms in front of his body, keeping the elbows extended.

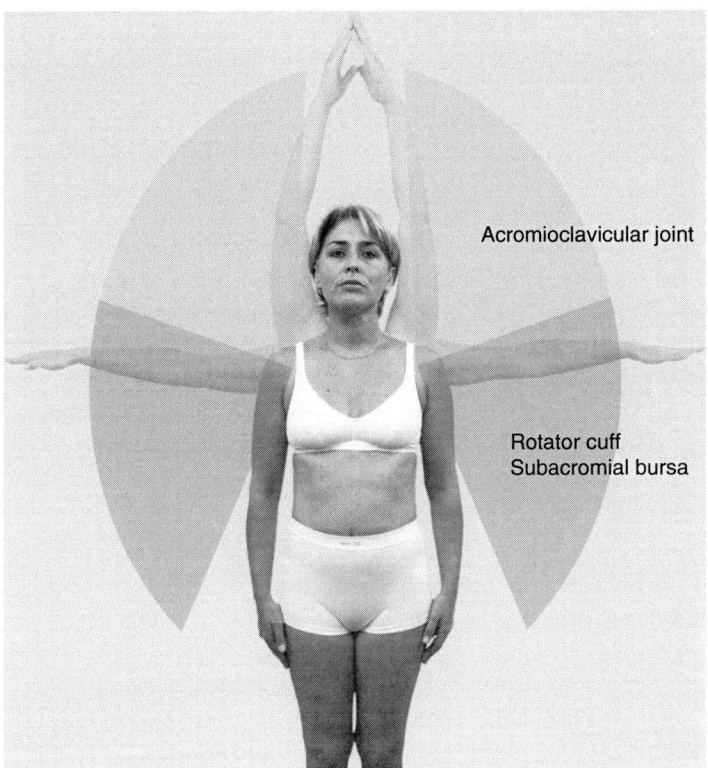

Acromioclavicular joint

Rotator cuff
Subacromial bursa

FIGURE 1.8 Clinical examination of the shoulder region: active abduction. Typical painful arcs

Pain while performing this movement suggests a lesion of the biceps. In this case, the pain is located to the anterior aspect of the shoulder and upper arm. Note, however, that pain with this movement may also be caused by tendonitis of the supraspinatus or subacromial bursitis.

c. We now go on to passive mobilization. Ask the patient to relax his arm in your hand. Gentle passive movements and the assurance that this will hurt less can help to achieve this.

Standing behind and to the side of the patient, hold his forearm and mobilize it slowly and carefully to complete abduction (Fig. 1.9a) and then complete flexion (Fig. 1.9b). Your other hand lies on the patient's shoulder to feel any snapping or crepitus.

To assess internal and external rotation, the shoulder is placed in 90° abduction, with the elbow also bent to 90°. The hand is then pulled upwards (external rotation) and downwards (internal rotation) (Fig. 1.10a and b)

Ask the patient how intense the pain is in comparison to that which he felt during active mobilization and assess the range of movement.

If the pain is significantly less intense than that felt during active movement, tendonitis is more likely – of the supraspinatus, if abduction is painful or of the biceps if flexion is most affected. In these cases, we can expect passive movements to show a full range, even though there may be some pain.

If, on the other hand, mobility is limited mechanically and not just by the pain, we should suspect an intrinsic lesion of the glenohumeral joint and/or its capsule. In this case, we can sometimes detect crepitus or snapping in the joint. In glenohumeral synovitis, all movements are generally painful.

In the presence of limited abduction, it is useful to assess the glenohumeral separately from the scapulothoracic component. To do this, stand behind the patient and hold the lower vertex of the scapula, following its movement while inducing abduction of the arm (Fig. 1.11). With the shoulder blade immobilized, a normal glenohumeral joint allows about 90° abduction.

Significant limitation of all movements is highly suggestive of adhesive capsulitis, especially if external rotation is limited. Most arthropathies limit abduction earlier, leaving rotation, and especially internal rotation, relatively free.

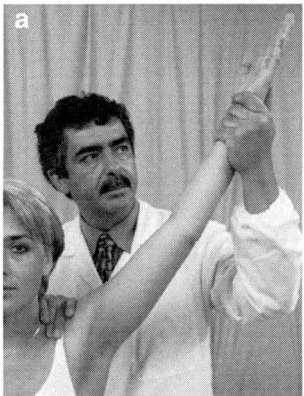

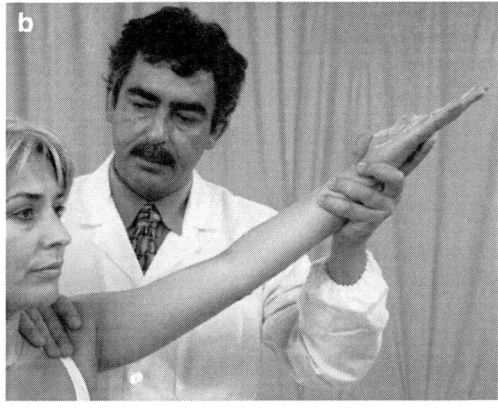

FIGURE 1.9 Passive mobilization of the shoulder. (**a**) Abduction. (**b**) Flexion. *Please note: the correct interpretation of passive motion demands that the patient is relaxed*

d. Resisted mobilization also requires an appropriate technique.

   i) The patient's arms are placed at 90° abduction and about 30° ahead of the frontal plane, with the thumbs turned down (The greater tuberosity is under the acromion). Ask the patient to hold this position while you push his forearms down (Fig. 1.12).

ii) The patient puts his hand on the opposite shoulder and raises his elbow until his arm is horizontal. He holds the position while you push his elbow down (Fig. 1.13).

iii) With the patient's shoulder at 90° abduction and 30° anterior flexion, the elbows are bent to 90°. You push the shoulder down while raising and internally rotating the arm with the other hand (Fig. 1.14 Subacromial conflict test).

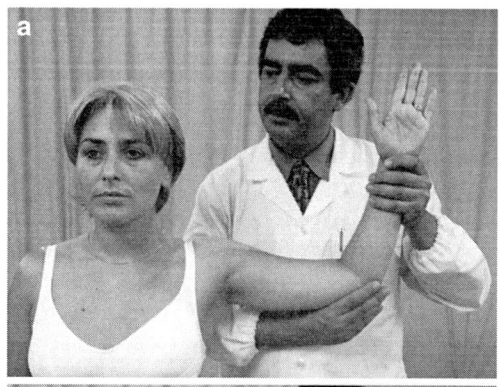

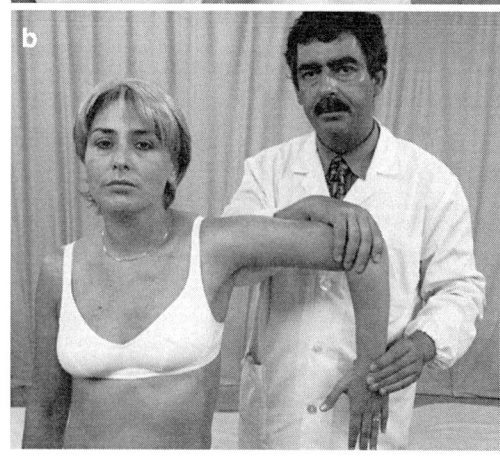

FIGURE 1.10 Passive mobilization of the shoulder. (**a**) External rotation. (**b**) Internal rotation

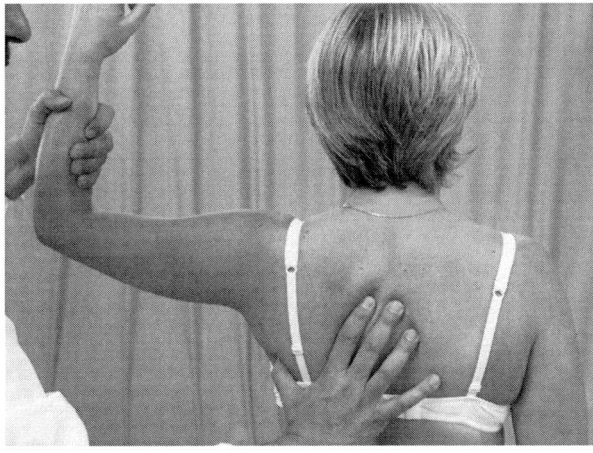

FIGURE 1.11 Precise evaluation of shoulder abduction due to the glenohumeral joint. Immobilization of the scapula precludes the scapulothoracic component

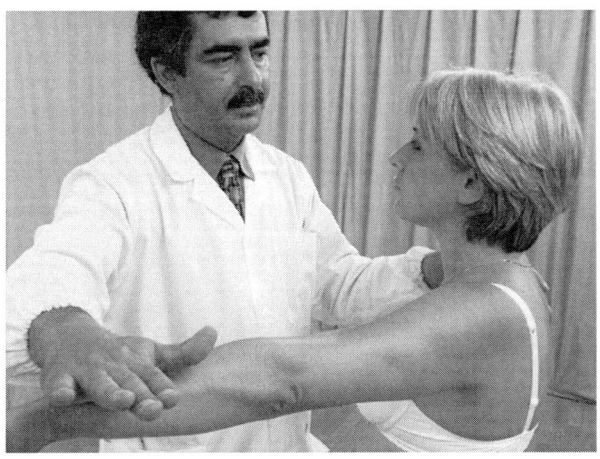

FIGURE 1.12 Resisted abduction of the shoulder. The rotator cuff (supra- and infraspinatus) is put under tension and the subacromial bursa is compressed

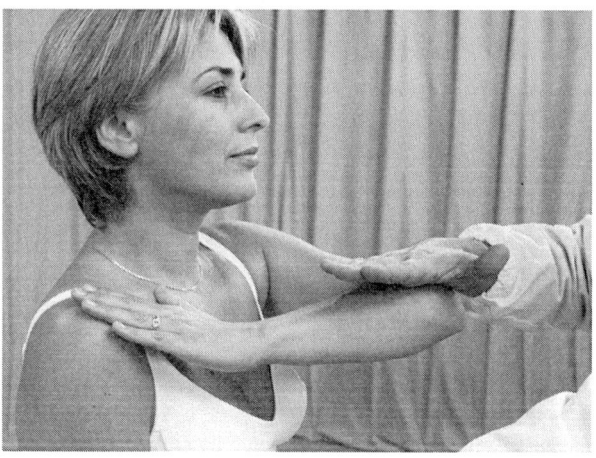

FIGURE 1.13 Subacromial impingement test. The rotator cuff (supra- and infraspinatus) is put under tension and the subacromial bursa is compressed

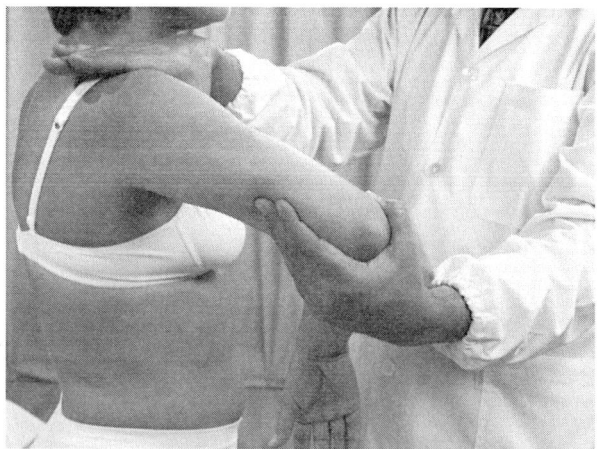

FIGURE 1.14 Subacromial impingement test

The first two maneuvers require contraction of the supraspinatus, placing its tendon under tension. In addition, this contraction pulls the head of the humerus up towards the acromion, compressing the rotator cuff and the subacromial bursa against it. In the third maneuver, the observer induces the movement. If there is any inflammation of the supraspinatus tendon or bursa, the patient will complain of pain in the shoulder region – a positive maneuver. When these maneuvers cause pain in locations other than the shoulder, we should suspect hyperreactivity to pain, as in fibromyalgia for example.

In practice, it is very difficult in a clinical examination to distinguish between tendonitis of the supraspinatus and subacromial bursitis. This is not particularly important as the treatment is very similar.

e. We then test the biceps.

  i. The patient raises his arms anteriorly to 30–45° flexion, with his elbows and wrists in extension and supination (Palms up test or Speed's test). He holds this position while you force his forearms down (Fig. 1.15).

  ii. The patient places his arm along his body, the elbow bent to 90° and the hand semi-supine. He holds this position, while resisting your efforts to extend his elbow and pronate the hand (Yergason's maneuver – Fig. 1.16).

The maneuvers are positive if they cause pain in the anterior aspect of the shoulder and proximal third of the upper arm, suggesting tenosynovitis of the long head of the biceps.

Palpation

As the shoulder is a deep joint, it is not possible to palpate the joint space or look for effusion. There are, however, two sites where palpation is particularly productive:

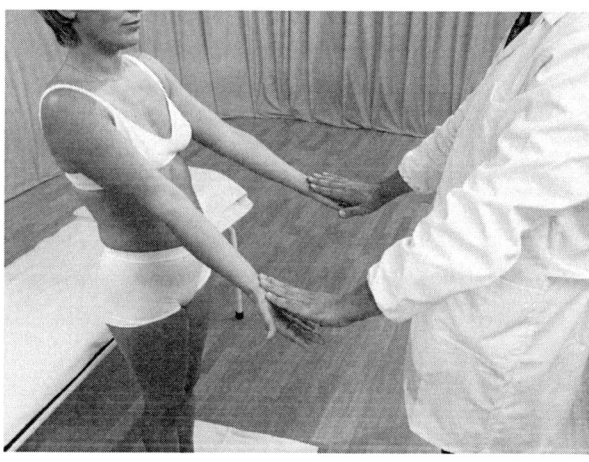

FIGURE 1.15 Palms up test (Speed's test). Pain in the shoulder suggests tenosynovitis of the long head of the biceps

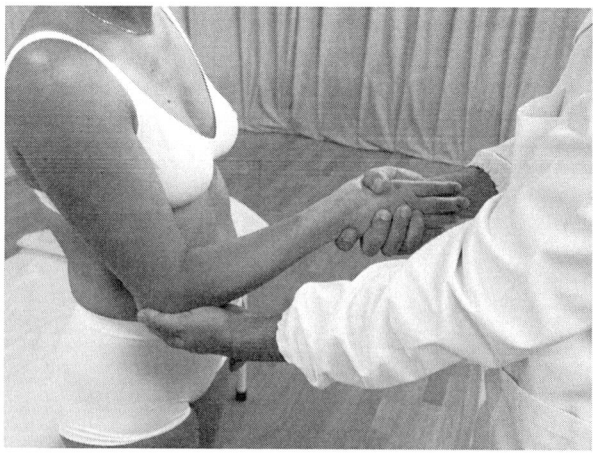

FIGURE 1.16 Yergason's test. The examiner tries to pronate and extend the forearm, while the patient resists. Pain in the shoulder suggests tenosynovitis of the long head of the biceps

Supraspinatus and infraspinatus tendon/subacromial bursa

With the arm at rest, they are the soft structures that you feel between the external border of the acromion, above, and the bony prominence of the greater tuberosity below (Fig. 1.17a). Alternatively, ask the patient to put his hand behind his back. This makes the greater tuberosity rotate forward to a position below and in front of the anterior vertex of the acromion (Fig. 1.17b).[2] Pain on deep palpation of these areas suggests a lesion of the supraspinatus or subacromial bursitis. If in doubt, compare with the other side.

Tendon of the long head of the biceps

To examine the tendon on the right side, stand behind and to the right of the patient and hold his forearm in your left hand. Run the fingertips of your right hand deeply across the head of the humerus. You will feel the greater and lesser tuberosities and the bicipital groove between them. If necessary, rotate the patient's shoulder inwards and outwards while you palpate. The tendon of the long head of the biceps and its sheath feel like a sinewy roll running along the groove and extending downwards. Local pain on palpation suggests tenosynovitis (Fig. 1.18).

---

[2] Try it on yourself. Place your right hand at rest along your body. Press the head of the humerus with your left index finger just below the anterior vertex of the right acromion. Now rotate your hand inwards and outwards – the bony prominence that you can feel deep down gliding under your finger is the greater tuberosity.

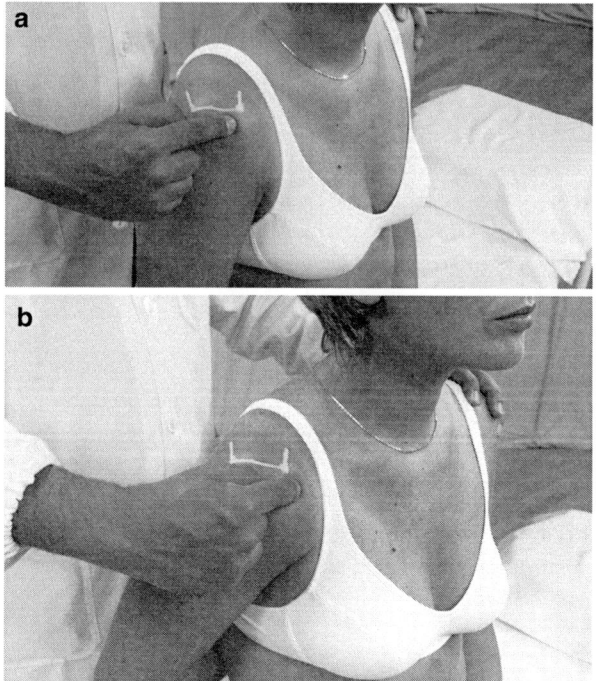

FIGURE 1.17 Palpation of the insertion of the rotator cuff in the greater tuberosity of the humerus, with the shoulder in neutral position (**a**) or in internal rotation (**b**)

Please note: As the glenohumeral joint is deeply located, it is difficult to absolutely confirm or exclude the existence of arthritis. We have to base our assessment on the rhythm of the pain, on the clinical context (monoarthritis of the shoulder is rare) and on passive mobilization: restriction of movements indicates a compromised joint. If the patient experiences pain during passive mobilization of the shoulder, rotating the arm to an angle of about 50°, there is probably inflammation of the synovium or capsule.

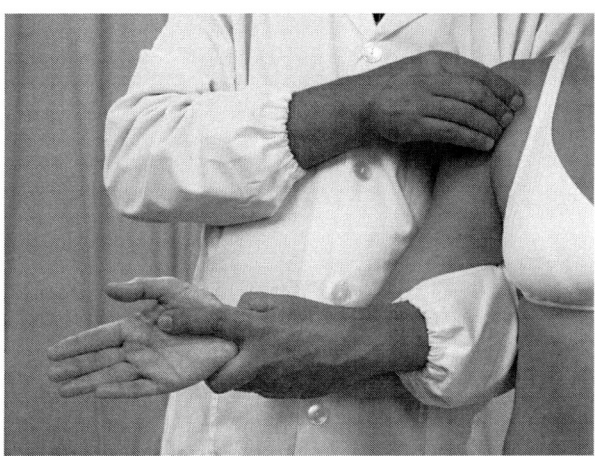

FIGURE 1.18 Palpation of tendon of the long head of the biceps. The tendon, surrounded by its synovial sheath, lies in the bicipital grove, on the anterior aspect of the humerus. It is easier to palpate while the shoulder is rotated internally and externally

Typical Cases
1.A. Shoulder Pain (I)

Mr. Figueiredo was a 48-year old draftsman. He was sent to us by his family doctor because of pain involving his right shoulder, which he had had for about 3 months. The pain troubled him particularly at night, stopping him lying on the right, his usual position. He felt no pain at rest, but movements caused intense pain, especially when putting on his jacket, washing his back, combing his hair or changing gear in the car. There was no significant morning stiffness.

He denied any recent or old trauma. He did not practice sport or have any special hobbies, but he spent a long time at the computer as part of his job. He mentioned sporadic, transient lumbar and cervical pain which he attributed to long hours sitting at the computer. He denied recent neck pain or paresthesia and said that moving his neck did not exacerbate the pain in his shoulder. He had no other symptoms or associated disease.

Think about the most probable causes of this pain.
Imagine you were the patient's doctor. How would you examine him?

A comparative inspection of the shoulders did not show any asymmetry. During the general rheumatologic examination, the patient complained of intense pain in his right shoulder during abduction, beginning at about 60° and with no relief on complete abduction. Anterior flexion of the arms caused some discomfort in the same area, though it was less intense. Passive mobilization of the shoulder in abduction caused pain, though it was much less severe than during active mobilization. The patient was anxious and unable to relax completely. Passive flexion of the shoulder was painless. The maneuvers of resisted abduction and resisted elevation of the arm with the hand on the opposite shoulder were painful. There was no significant pain in the palms up test or Yergason's maneuver. Palpation over the greater tuberosity of the humerus was very painful compared to the other side, particularly with the arm in internal rotation. The examination of the cervical spine and elbow was normal.

Summarize this condition.[3]
What is your diagnosis?
Do we need diagnostic tests? Which ones?
What treatment would you choose?
In view of the ineffectiveness of previous measures, we injected a mixture of local anesthetic and methylprednisolone around the supraspinatus tendon and the subacromial space. The patient experienced considerable relief when we repeated active mobilization a few minutes later, which

_____

[3]A young patient with selective shoulder pain – pain worse during active than passive mobilization, without range limitations. Rotator cuff maneuvers positive.

confirmed our diagnosis: supraspinatus tendonitis/subacromial bursitis.

We explained to the patient the cause of his pain and his anatomical condition. We said that the situation was highly likely to recur as, in most cases, it is related to a constitutional subacromial space conflict. We advised him to avoid repeated work with his arms raised above his shoulders and suggested that it would be a very good idea to use supports for his forearms when working at the computer. We told him to come back if the pain persisted. After 6 months we still had not seen him, but we would not be surprised if he came back with similar problems.

Supraspinatus Tendonitis and Subacromial Bursitis
Main Points

This is a very common condition in adults and the elderly.

When it appears in young people we should suspect glenohumeral instability.

The pain is usually unilateral and limited to the shoulder, rarely radiating to the arm. It is highly incapacitating.

As a rule, the pain is more intense during abduction than during flexion of the shoulder. It may be worse at night, especially lying on the same side.

Although it is usually an isolated problem, it may be associated with arthritis of the shoulder or other soft tissue lesions, especially tenosynovitis of the biceps.

A careful clinical examination usually provides the diagnosis.

Diagnostic tests are not necessary in typical cases, as they have nothing to add to the diagnosis or the choice of treatment.

Initial treatment is conservative, with topical and systemic anti-inflammatories and local protection.

In persistent or highly incapacitating cases, a local injection of glucocorticoids by an experienced professional is justified and usually solves the problem.

It is highly likely to recur and in exceptional cases may warrant surgery.

Typical Cases

1.B. Frozen Shoulder

Isabel dos Santos was a 62-year old farm worker. She came to our clinic because of pain and lack of mobility in the right shoulder, for which she had been on sick leave for the last 7 weeks. The pain was constant day and night and worsened with any attempt at movement. It was partially relieved by anti-inflammatories, but they did nothing for the limited mobility. When she first experienced these symptoms, she was sent for physiotherapy. The pain was exacerbated by mobilization, even when passive, however, and she refused any more treatment after a few sessions. She had been given an injection in the upper aspect of the shoulder. She had noticed no improvement.

When asked about trauma, she said that she had had a fall at work a few days before the shoulder pain appeared but that she had recovered immediately. She was being treated regularly for hypertension and diabetes, both of which were under control, and denied any other symptoms. She had undergone the menopause, spontaneously at 42. Her mother had been healthy and had died at the age of 82 as a result of a hip fracture.

Her clinical examination was normal. She was 1.48 m tall and weighed 45 kg.

Our general rheumatologic examination showed atrophy of the right shoulder muscles. The joint was almost completely immobilized and extremely painful. When asked to abduct her shoulder, the patient leaned her body to the left and only managed to raise her shoulder to about 40° abduction. Passive mobilization was extremely painful and highly limited in all directions, including internal and external rotation. On immobilizing the scapula, we found that almost all abduction was due to swinging the scapula. There were no anomalies in the cervical spine or the rest of the rheumatologic examination, apart from moderate dorsal kyphosis.

Frozen Shoulder, Adhesive Capsulitis of the Shoulder
Main Points

This is a relatively uncommon, but highly incapacitating condition that can leave important sequelae if not treated properly.

It is an inflammatory, fibrosing process that affects the articular capsule and causes it to contract over the joint, thus limiting its mobility. Loss of external rotation is particularly suggestive of this condition.

The pain tends to be intense and constant, especially in the early stages of the disease, getting worse at night and with movement. It may subside spontaneously after a few weeks or months.

Limited active and passive mobility in all directions is an essential clinical clue. It may be the only manifestation in the late stages.

It may appear spontaneously, but there is often a history of trauma (even very small). Repeated tendonitis of the cuff, previous stroke and diabetes mellitus are predisposing factors.

Diagnostic tests serve essentially to rule out other pathologies like septic arthritis, intra-articular fracture, or aseptic necrosis of the humerus. In adhesive capsulitis, the standard x-ray of the shoulder is normal. Arthrography, CT scans and ultrasound can be used to confirm the diagnosis.

Although intra-articular injection of corticosteroids may be difficult, it helps to relieve the pain if administered in the initial stages of the condition.

Physiotherapy and regular exercise at home, together with analgesics and anti-inflammatories, play an essential role in restoring mobility, which may take up to 2 years.

In rare cases, recovery may require manipulation of the shoulder under anesthetic to break down the fibrosis, followed by physiotherapy.

What do you think are the most likely diagnoses?
Would you ask for any diagnostic tests?
What treatment would you suggest in each case?

In view of the symptoms, we thought the most probable diagnosis was adhesive capsulitis. We asked for a full blood count, sedimentation rate and anteroposterior x-rays in a neutral position and arranged to see her again soon. All these tests were normal. There were no signs of fracture or changes in the bone structure of the humeral head or articular space of the right glenohumeral joint, when compared to the left.

We gave her an intra-articular injection of a long-acting corticosteroid, using an anterior approach to the joint. We noted considerable resistance to the pressure of the injection. We told the patient that we expected her pain to be greatly relieved and stressed the need for intense, prolonged physiotherapy. She would have to do regular exercises at home to increase the range of movement. We pointed out that complete recovery of mobility could take up to 2 years. We prescribed an anti-inflammatory for which she had already shown good tolerance, to take when necessary for the pain. We scheduled follow-up visits to assess mobility, which we recorded with a goniometer, for future reference.

Reconsider the case. Have we forgotten anything, like additional tests?[4]

Consider the possible causes and their likelihood.

List the maneuvers that you think are necessary and their interpretation.

Typical Cases
1.C. Shoulder Pain (II)
António Rodrigues, a 43-year old stonemason, complained of pain in his left shoulder that had started 2 months before, after a particularly strenuous job. The pain was diffuse, but

---

[4]In fact, we also looked for osteoporosis. This is a typical situation in which we should consider this condition as there are a number of risk factors: post-menopausal woman with an early menopause, underweight and a family history suggesting the disease.

was more marked on the anterior aspect of the shoulder. He said that he had trouble picking up heavy weights and often dropped them because of the pain. Other movements were fairly easy. He denied any pain at night or at rest.

He was otherwise healthy with no other musculoskeletal or systemic complaints.

Our general examination did not find any anomalies. Active mobilization of the shoulder was complete and painless. The maneuvers for the rotator cuff were only slightly uncomfortable. The palms-up-test caused typical pain, however. Yergason's maneuver was also painful. Palpation of the left bicipital groove was much more painful than the right.

What is your diagnosis?
How would you treat it?
We diagnosed tenosynovitis of the long head of the right biceps.

We explained the situation to the patient, and suggested a period of rest, if possible with his arm in a sling. We prescribed anti-inflammatories, and scheduled a new appointment for a local injection if the situation did not clear up completely in 3 or 4 weeks.

Imagine you are a general practitioner. What possible diagnoses do you think are likely? Why?
Would you request any diagnostic tests?

Tenosynovitis of the Long Head of the Biceps
Main Points
This is a common condition in adults and the elderly.

The pain is usually unilateral and confined to the anterior face of the shoulder. It may be highly incapacitating.

As a rule, the pain is more intense on flexion of the shoulder. There may be nocturnal pain.

Although it is usually isolated, it can be associated with arthritis of the shoulder or other soft tissue lesions, especially supraspinatus tendonitis.

A careful clinical examination usually provides the diagnosis.

Diagnostic tests are not necessary in typical cases, as they have nothing to add to the diagnosis or the choice of treatment.

Initial treatment is conservative, with topical and systemic anti-inflammatories and local protection.

In persistent or highly incapacitating cases, local injection by an experienced physician is indicated.

Typical Cases
1.D. Shoulder Pain (III)

António Sarmento was a 46-year old salesman. He came to us because of a deep, "dull" ache in his left shoulder, which was difficult to pinpoint and had started about 8 months before. The pain came in episodes and went away by itself after several minutes to 1 hour. He did not recognize a clear trigger for the pain, but he noticed it was related to more demanding physical activities, particularly climbing stairs. He attributed a curiously distressing character to it. It was sometimes associated with discomfort over the lower part of the sternum. He had been treated with anti-inflammatories to no avail.

Our systematic enquiry revealed no other alterations. He smoked about 30 cigarettes a day and was not taking any regular medication.

The patient was obese and good-humored. Our clinical and general rheumatologic examinations showed no alterations except hypertension (160/95 mmHg). Movements of both shoulders were free and painless, both on passive and active mobilization. Periarticular palpation was painless. The examination of the cervical spine was also normal, causing no pain in the shoulder. Auscultation of the heart and lungs showed no anomalies.

On the basis of this information, we requested routine tests with an evaluation of serum lipids. His ECG showed slight elevation of the ST segment in the left precordial leads. After this finding the patient did an exercise test, which was positive, with clear signs of coronary ischemia coinciding with the pain in his shoulder, similar to that described spontaneously. The patient was referred to a cardiologist for a possible coronary angiography. When we saw him again about 3 months later he was asymptomatic following introduction of nitrates.

He's your patient! What other questions would you ask him?

Referred Shoulder Pain
Main Points

Pain of cervical, coronary, pleural and subdiaphragmatic origin can radiate to the shoulder.

This pain is ill-defined and variable, depending on the cause.

A careful systematic enquiry can produce suggestive clues.

Regional clinical examination is normal.

An examination of the neck may show alterations and reproduce the pain, suggesting a cervical origin.

The treatment is oriented by the underlying cause.

Typical Cases
1.E. Shoulder Pain (IV)

Carlos Soares, a 52-year old carpenter, decided to go to the doctor after many years of pain in both shoulders, because the symptoms were worsening and his functional disability was progressive. The pain had begun 10–12 years previously, and had continued since then with exacerbations and partial remissions. A workaholic, he attributed the pain to his occupation and continued to work in spite of everything, taking anti-inflammatories when it got worse. Now this was no longer possible. The pain in his right shoulder was incapacitating and its mobility was greatly reduced.

When asked, he also described a history of low back pain that had begun at the same time, with similar progression and characteristics: more intense when the work was harder. However, he also had pain at night and mentioned morning stiffness of the shoulder and lumbar region lasting about an hour.

He denied any systemic manifestations and his past medical history was not relevant.

Plan the main points of a clinical examination of this patient.

In the general clinical examination, we found obvious scaly erythematous lesions dispersed over the torso and scalp (Fig. 1.19), which the patient said he had had for years though it did not bother him.

Mobility of the lumbar spine seemed reduced and Schober's test showed an elongation of 10–12.5 cm.

Mobility in his right shoulder was considerably reduced, limited to 120° abduction and 90° anterior flexion. Internal and external rotation were also reduced. Passive mobilization did not increase these ranges and was accompanied by moderate pain in all directions. The maneuvers for periarticular lesions were negative. There were no other alterations in the rest of the examination.

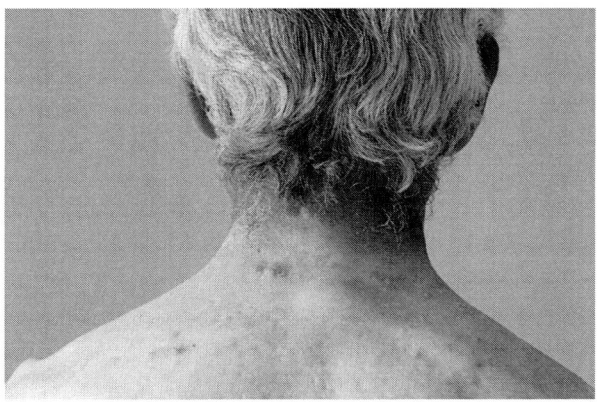

FIGURE 1.19 Erythematous and scaling lesions – psoriasis

Summarize this clinical case.[5]
What are the most probable diagnoses?
Would you ask for any diagnostic tests?
What treatment would you prescribe?
We requested lab tests, including a full blood count, sedimentation rate, liver and kidney tests, and x-rays of the shoulders (anteroposterior in neutral position and with external rotation), pelvis (anteroposterior) and lumbar spine (anteroposterior and profile). The tests showed a discreet elevation of the sedimentation rate to 32 mm in the first hour with no other alterations. The radiograph of the shoulders showed diffuse osteopenia on the right, reduction of the joint space with some sclerosis of the articular surfaces and osteophyte formations (Fig. 1.20a). The x-ray of the pelvis showed sclerosis and partial blurring of the right sacroiliac joint (second degree sacroiliitis – Fig. 1.20b).

---

[5]Inflammatory shoulder and back pain in a patient with psoriasis. Limited active and passive mobility in the painful areas.

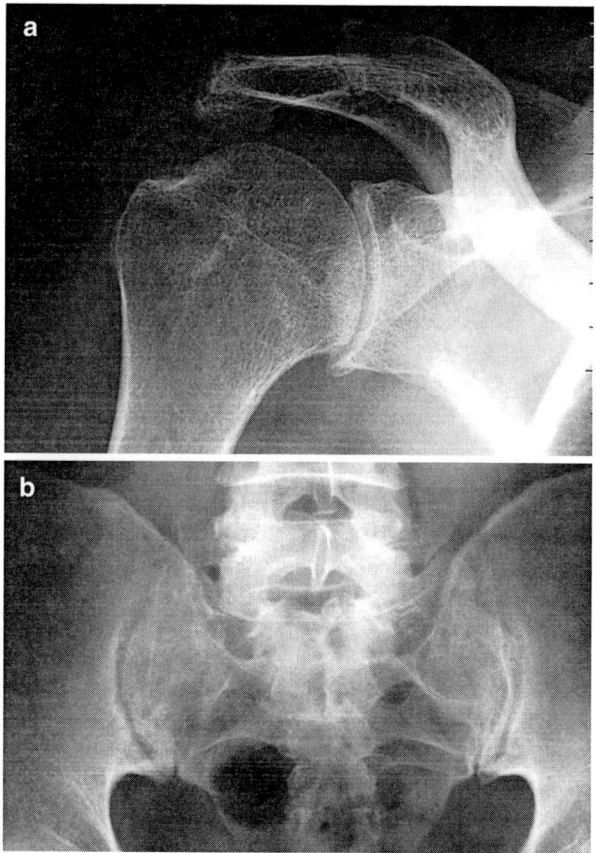

FIGURE 1.20 (**a**) Radiology of the shoulder – advanced arthritis. Note the joint space loss, diffuse osteopenia, displacement superiorly of the humeral head and osteophytes in the periphery of the glenoid surface. (**b**) The X-rays of the pelvis revealed subchondral sclerosis, erosions and partial blurring of the right sacroiliac joint

Inflammatory Shoulder Pain
Main Points
The shoulder can be involved in practically all types of polyarthritis.

Even when the complaints are focused in one area, it is essential to ask about other joints.

The inflammatory rhythm of the pain, an important clue to diagnosis, may be difficult to pinpoint, especially in manual workers.

Clinical examination is fundamental to the diagnosis. Pain on passive mobilization in several directions and limited active and passive mobility indicate joint disease.

Without proper treatment, arthritis can leave irreversible sequelae.

Treatment should begin early and be suited to the nature of the disease.

We considered that this confirmed the diagnosis of psoriatic arthritis, with involvement of the sacroiliac joints and the right shoulder, with secondary osteoarthritis of this joint and persistent inflammatory activity. It was unfortunate that the patient's joint disease was so advanced when he came to us.

The patient was advised to try to spare his shoulder as much as possible. We prescribed a long-lasting anti-inflammatory, to be taken with the evening meal, supplemented during the day, if necessary. We suggested regular exercises for both the affected regions. We recommended an intra-articular injection of the shoulder, which was highly effective. The patient was kept under clinical observation, saving further therapy for the involvement of any other articular areas.

Special Situations

Joint Disease and Instability of the Acromioclavicular Joint

Instability of the acromioclavicular joint is usually the result of trauma, such as a fall onto the outstretched arm. This joint can be involved in inflammatory arthropathies of several types.

Osteoarthritis may appear as a result of repeated trauma, usually from heavy manual labor. The pain is usually felt on the upper surface of the shoulder. Active mobilization causes pain in extreme movements in all directions and pain arising above 90° abduction is especially typical. The joint is accessible to local palpation, which may detect inflammatory or bony swelling and instability.

The most specific maneuver for examining this joint involves asking the patient to put one hand behind his back, with his elbow in extension. We then force adduction to the limit. The presence of acromioclavicular lesion is suggested by pain over the joint.

Instability and Subluxation of the Gleno-Humeral Joint

This usually appears in young people, especially athletes, after violent movements like throwing a ball. It presents acutely with a "dead-arm" sensation, with intense pain, numbness and tingling in the arm, followed by a deeper pain. It is often followed by rotator cuff tendonitis for a few days or weeks. It has a marked tendency to recur, which is accentuated by repeated episodes of dislocation, even if each episode often resolves spontaneously.

In the presence of dislocation, there is a clear asymmetry of the shoulders on observation. To test stability, ask the patient to lie down with his upper limb hanging beside the examining table. Then immobilize the shoulder with one hand and hold the arm with the other. With the patient relaxed, try to induce anterior and posterior movements of the head of the humerus, noting the degree of instability and comparing it to the opposite side if necessary (Fig. 1.21a). Another way of testing stability consists of forcing external rotation and anterior projection of the humerus, while the arm is abducted to 90° (Fig. 1.21b). This maneuver assesses anterior instability and is positive if there is pain or a sensation of anterior dislocation of the head of the humerus. If posterior compression of the shoulder relieves this pain, this reinforces the suggestion of instability.

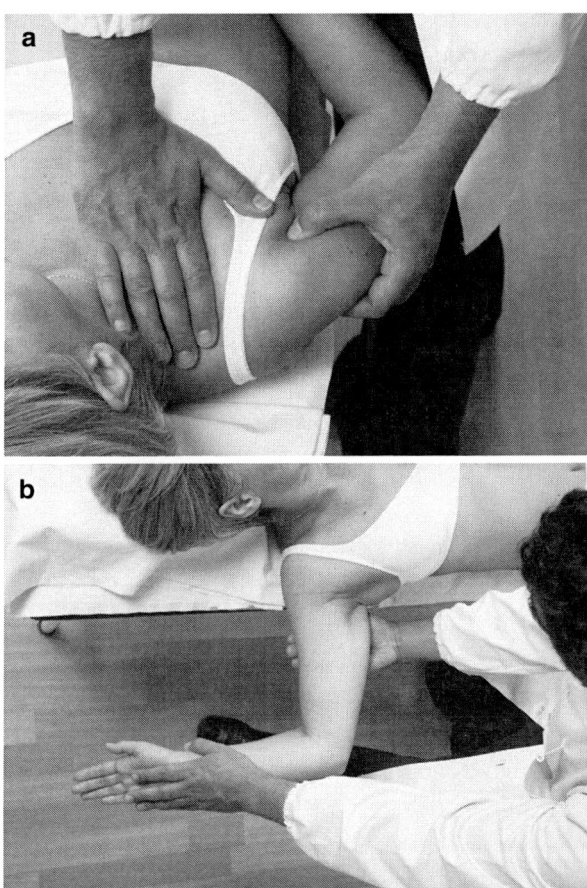

FIGURE 1.21 Shoulder stability test. (**a**) The hand holding the upper arm tests the antero-posterior mobility at the joint level. The other stabilizes the collar bone and the acromion. (**b**) The external rotation with anterior projection of the humerus causes pain. The diagnosis is reinforced if the pain subsides with posterior projection of the head of the humerus

This suspicion justifies referring the patient to a special rehabilitation program.

Acute Shoulder

Acute shoulder pain, sometimes accompanied by swelling, suggests trauma, infection or micro-crystalline joint disease. Septic arthritis of the shoulder is rare but highly destructive and requires early treatment. Chondrocalcinosis and the deposit of hydroxyapatite crystals may result in acute, sometimes rapidly destructive arthritis.

These situations require urgent referral for diagnostic tests (joint aspirate, for example) and treatment. Stabilizing surgical procedures, preferably arthroscopic, are sometimes necessary.

Diagnostic Tests

Diagnostic tests are dispensable in most patients with regional shoulder pain. The enquiry and clinical examination will reveal diagnostic characteristics of soft tissue lesion: selectivity of painful movements, unlimited passive mobility that is less painful than active movement, resisted mobilization, and local palpation.

Some tests may be justified in cases of signs or symptoms suggesting joint disease or unclear, persistent clinical conditions.

Imaging

A ***standard x-ray*** of the shoulder is more productive in cases of joint disease and can show the typical characteristics of inflammatory or degenerative disease (Fig. 1.20a). It sometimes shows the presence of calcifications of the supraspinatus tendon or the subacromial bursa – calcifying tendonitis

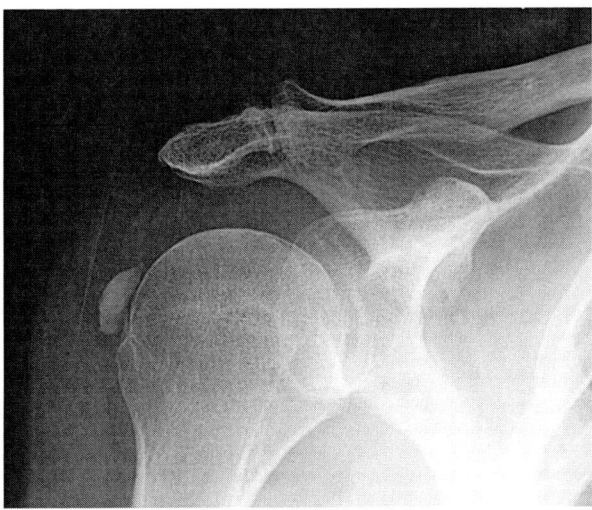

FIGURE 1.22 Subacromial calcification. Calcifying tendonitis or bursitis

(Fig. 1.22). Although this finding will not alter the treatment, it indicates a chronic, recurring lesion, which is more resistant to conservative treatment. In some cases, we can see sclerosis and irregularity of the greater tuberosity, which indicates a similar pathology. X-rays can also show fractures and lytic lesions.

Ultrasound scans are more useful in soft tissue lesions and in experienced hands can detect inflammatory lesions or tears and pinpoint their exact location.

CT and MRI scans can make a valuable contribution to clearing up complex cases in specialized investigations.

Other Tests

Lab tests are indicated if there is reason to suspect inflammatory joint disease and are selected according to the nature of the joint disease suggested by the clinical evaluation. Changes in the full blood count and sedimentation rate are non-specific clues to inflammatory joint disease. Liver and kidney tests may be justified especially in preparation for possible disease-modifying treatment. Tests for rheumatoid factor are justified if the clinical assessment suggests rheumatoid arthritis. Suspected septic arthritis (acute/subacute monoarthritis, fever and leukocytosis) justifies referring the patient immediately to a specialized centre.

Treatment

Most cases of regional shoulder pain correspond to soft tissue lesions and simple measures should be taken, as described above.

In the case of joint disease, which is potentially highly incapacitating, the patient should be sent to a specialist.

1. *Educating the patient*. Periarthritis of the shoulder is often related to an anatomical predisposition and repetitive work or leisure-related movements. As a result, they are highly likely to recur. Patients should be told this and taught how to avoid high-risk activities. They should be encouraged to take progressive, regular exercise as soon as the acute pain phase passes.
2. *Medication*. Anti-inflammatories, chosen according to the patient's particular condition, generally achieve marked relief of the pain. They can be aided by topical anti-inflammatories applied as a cream or patch several times a day in association with local heat.

   In highly incapacitating cases or those that have resisted prior treatment, local (intra- or periarticular) injection of an anesthetic and corticosteroid may be useful. These measures serve not only to confirm the diagnosis, but are also often effective in treating the condition itself. This kind of injection requires experience and a precise technique. In very advanced joint disease or ruptured tendons, performing a nerve block around the suprascapular nerve as it runs along the suprascapular groove may relieve the symptoms and improve mobility.

3. *Physiotherapy.* This is particularly useful in cases of persistent limitation of mobility, if the x-ray shows no signs of advanced, irreversible destruction of the joint structure. It is indispensable in cases of adhesive capsulitis.

   The use of physical agents like deep heat and microwaves can be beneficial in cases of soft tissue lesions that are resistant to simpler measures.

4. *Surgery.* This is limited to situations that have resisted the above treatments. In cases of recurring subacromial lesion with a conflict of space, the surgeon may use subacromial decompression with acromioplasty and removal of the coracoacromial ligament, which can be done arthroscopically. A shoulder prosthesis may be necessary in cases of great functional disability with irreversible structural damage of the glenohumeral joint. The results are better when surgery is carried out at specialized centers.

When should the Patient be Referred to a Specialist?

Whenever passive mobility of the joint is significantly limited.

When x-rays show obvious alterations in the joint or bone.

Whenever shoulder pain is associated with confirmed or suspected arthritis (mono-, oligo- or polyarthritis). Suspected septic arthritis requires urgent referral.

When conservative measures prove ineffective, with continued significant suffering and disability.

Chapter 2
Regional Syndromes
The Elbow and Forearm

The elbow is a complex joint. Its great functional importance derives from its involvement in the positioning and optimizing use of the hand. Elbow pain is usually superficial and localized, often radiating to the forearm. It is exacerbated by exercise such as carrying heavy items or making a fist. Periarticular lesions are much more common than joint disease. The elbow may be involved in polyarthritis, but it rarely starts there. Osteoarthritis of the elbow is very rare.

Differential diagnosis is essentially clinical.

Functional Anatomy

The elbow combines three bones in three joints: the humeroradial, laterally, the humeroulnar, medially, and the proximal radioulnar joint. The humeroulnar joint conducts and limits flexion and extension. The other two joints are involved mainly in supination and pronation of the forearm and hand. When fully extended, the axis of the forearm and arm form a lateral angle (in valgus) of 5° (in men) to 15° (in women), which is lost when the elbow is in complete flexion.

A single capsule surrounds these three joints forming a voluminous recess at the extensor surface (Fig. 2.1). If there is accumulation of articular fluid or synovitis this is expelled during full extension, causing a palpable bulge around the olecranon, particularly on the medial side.

J.A.P. da Silva, A.D. Woolf, *Rheumatology of the Upper Limbs in Clinical Practice*, DOI 10.1007/978-1-4471-2242-5_2,

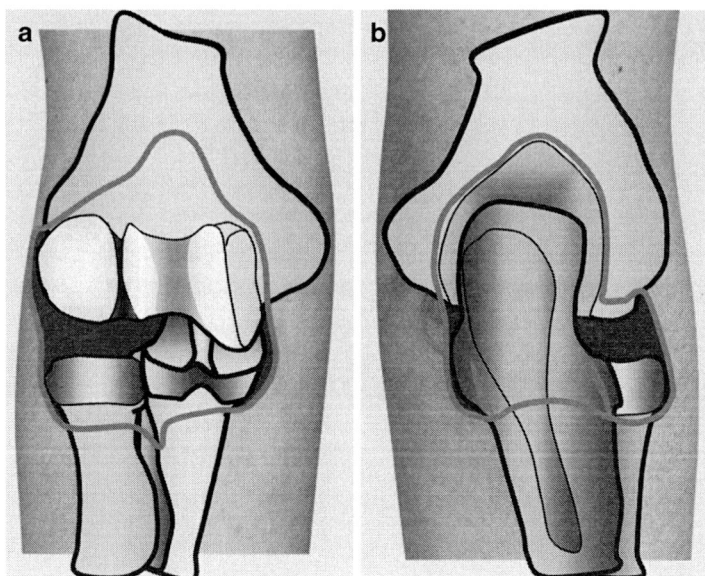

FIGURE 2.1 The elbow joints. The *green line* indicates the capsule insertion

Immediately above the articular surfaces of the humerus are two bony protrusions whose identification is of the greatest clinical importance: the lateral and medial epicondyles.[1]

Tendons are inserted at the lower border of these protrusions. These tendons are the most common sites of pathology in the elbow: lateral (tennis elbow) and medial epicondylitis (golfer's elbow). The extensors of the forearm and wrist insert into the lateral epicondyle and the flexors insert into the medial epicondyle (Fig. 2.2).

---

[1]Find these references in your own elbow. With your arm slightly bent, palpate the external border of the distal end of the humerus. You will feel the protrusion of the epicondyle and, under it, a rounded structure – the radial head. The epitrochlea is in the same location on the inside, but is more prominent. The tendons of flexor and extensor muscles of the hand are inserted along the lower surface of these protrusions.

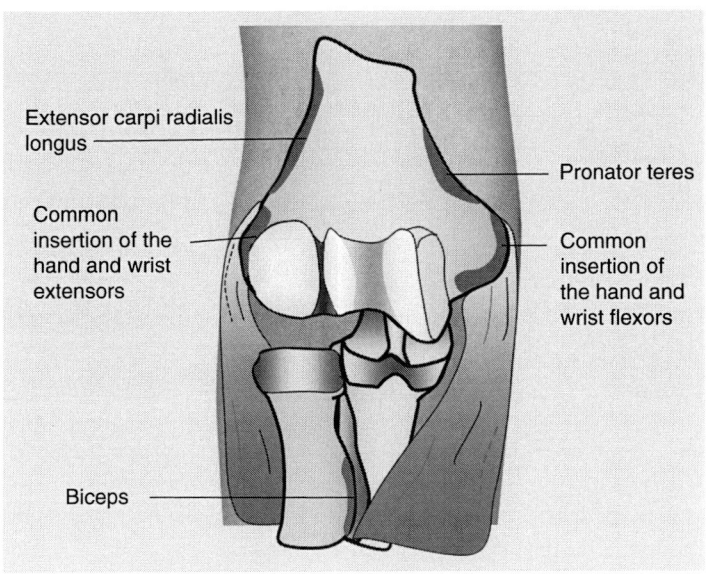

Extensor carpi radialis longus

Pronator teres

Common insertion of the hand and wrist extensors

Common insertion of the hand and wrist flexors

Biceps

FIGURE 2.2 Muscle insertions around the elbow joint

The elbow joint is served by a highly complex set of muscles. Extension is mediated by the triceps brachialis muscle, which joins the scapula and proximal humerus to the proximal end of the ulna (olecranon process). Elbow flexion is the result of the contraction of the biceps, (which joins the scapula to the radial tuberosity), the brachialis and the brachioradialis. Supination and pronation depend on specific muscles: the pronator teres, pronator quadratus, biceps and supinator.

The olecranon bursa covers the olecranon. It does not communicate with the joint, but is often the site of inflammation and effusion.

There are three other important points of reference.

- The ulnar nerve lies on the medial aspect, behind the medial epicondyle, in a tunnel consisting of branches of the humeroulnar ligament and the flexor carpi ulnaris. The ulnar nerve is easily entrapped along this route causing *ulnar nerve syndrome.*

FIGURE 2.3 Tender
point in the pronator
syndrome

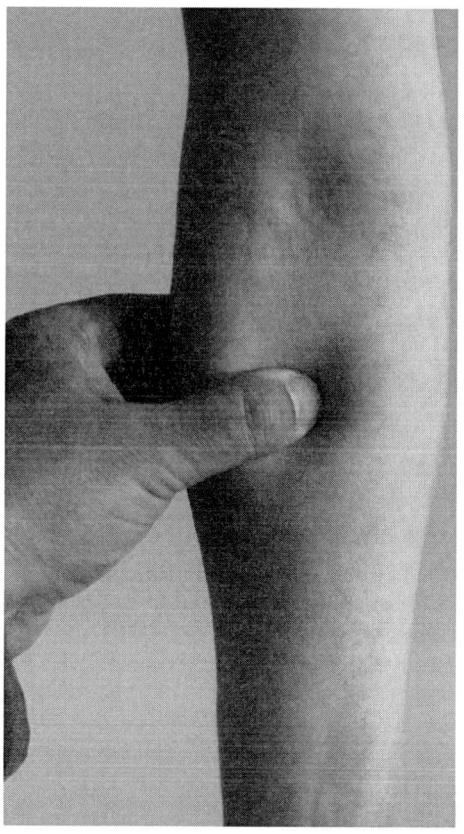

- The anterior interosseous nerve, a branch of the median
  nerve, emerges between the two parts of the pronator teres,
  at the mid-point of the union between the upper and middle
  third of the anterior aspect of the forearm (Fig. 2.3).
  Compression of this nerve branch can cause pain in the forearm (*pronator syndrome*).
- In about 30% of people, the posterior interosseous nerve, a
  branch of the radial nerve, passes between the two parts of
  the supinator on the posterolateral surface of the forearm
  (about 5 cm below the epicondyle – Fig. 2.4). Local compression of this nerve can cause *radial tunnel syndrome*.

FIGURE 2.4 Tender
point in the radial
tunnel syndrome

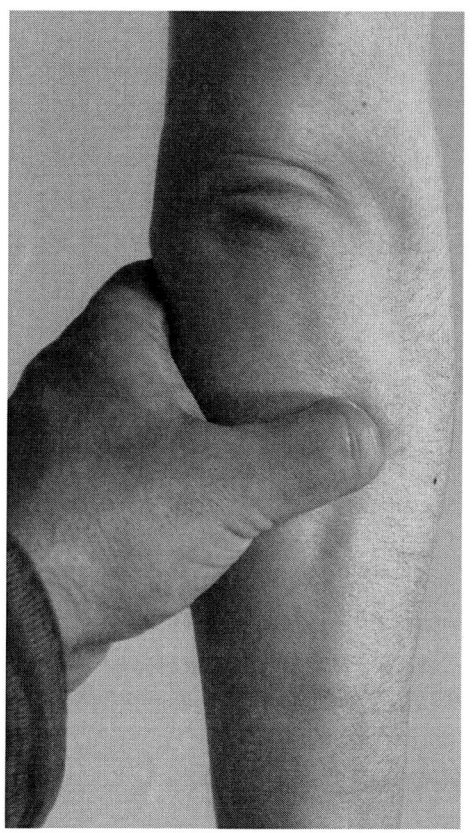

FIGURE 2.4 Tender point in the radial tunnel syndrome

Radiological Anatomy

From an anteroposterior view (Fig. 2.5) note the size and regularity of the humeroradial, humeroulnar and radioulnar articular space and the regularity and density of the articular surfaces. The epicondyles may show erosion or calcification. The lateral view (Fig. 2.6) is not so clear. Look at the humeroradial joint and the regularity of the olecranon.

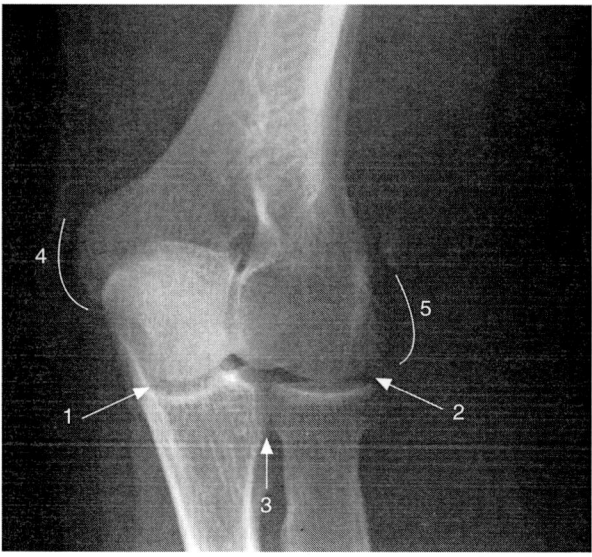

FIGURE 2.5 Normal radiology of the elbow. Left side antero-posterior view in extension, *1* Humeroulnar joint, *2* Humeroradial joint, *3* Superior radioulnar joint, *4* Medial epicondyle, *5* Lateral epicondyle

Common Causes of Pain in the Elbow and Forearm

Table 2.1 shows the most common causes of pain in the elbow and forearm.

The Enquiry

The first thing we should do is to check that the problem is actually limited to this area and does not affect any other joints or areas, suggesting polyarthropathy or generalized pain.

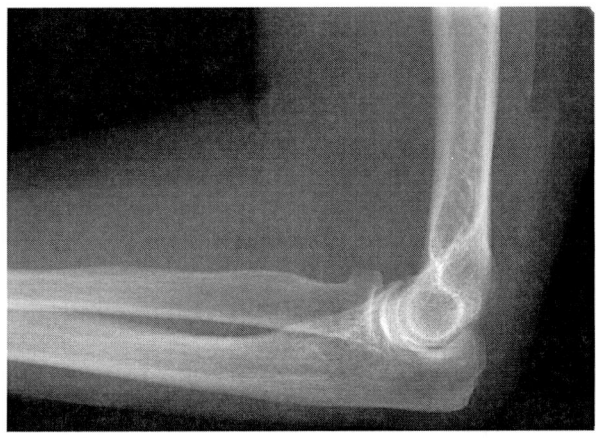

FIGURE 2.6 Radiology of the elbow. Lateral view. Note the radio-humeral joint space and the regularity of the olecranon

TABLE 2.1 Common causes of pain in the elbow and forearm

Etiology	Clinical clues
Lateral epicondylitis (Tennis elbow)	Pain at the lateral aspect of the elbow and forearm Worsens with extension of the wrist Pain on local palpation
Medial epicondylitis (Golfer's elbow)	Pain at the medial aspect of the elbow and forearm Worsens with flexion of the wrist Pain on local palpation
Olecranon bursitis	Pain at the vertex of the elbow Local swelling and tenderness
Trauma	History of trauma
Arthritis	Inflammatory pain Painful limitation of active and passive movements Posteromedial swelling
Referred pain	Pathology of the shoulder, neck, heart Local examination normal

In cases of tendonitis, the patient usually pinpoints the maximum pain on the medial or lateral aspect of the elbow. This pain often involves the same aspect of the forearm, sometimes as far as the distal third. Pain in tendonitis is usually exacerbated by exercise using the arm and forearm, such as carrying heavy items in the hands, or work involving flexion or extension of the wrist and fingers. The patient's work and leisure activities should be considered, as repetitive use is one of the main causes of these lesions.

Olecranon bursitis is normally obvious on local examination. It may be caused by repeated trauma (e.g. office workers), crystals (e.g. urate in gout) or infection. In other cases it is part of polyarthritis (e.g. rheumatoid arthritis).

Isolated arthritis of the elbow is rare and usually due to trauma or infection, but this joint is often involved in all types of polyarthritis. Osteoarthritis of the elbow is also rare. The type of pain, the clinical context and the physical examination are the basis of the diagnosis.

The presence of dysesthetic characteristics – burning sensation, electric shock, or tingling – should raise the possibility of radiculopathy or peripheral nerve compression – ulnar nerve syndrome. Sometimes, the symptoms caused by compression of the median nerve in the carpal tunnel radiate proximally, to the forearm.

Entrapment of the anterior or posterior interosseous nerves is relatively rare. It causes deep, undefined, persistent pain relatively unrelated to exercise, located respectively on the anterior and posterior aspect of the forearm. Curiously, the usual dysesthetic characteristics are often absent, although there may be paresthesia in the area of the median or radial nerve. When confronted with deep pain in the forearm, we should consider this possibility and conduct our physical examination accordingly (see below).

The forearm may be affected by pain radiating proximally from carpal tunnel syndrome, de Quervain 's tenosynovitis or wrist arthropathy, though the symptoms are predominantly in the wrist and hand.

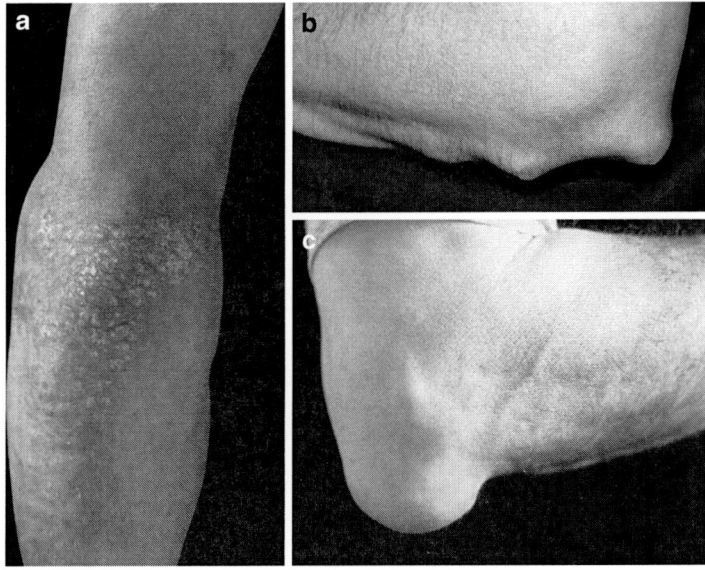

FIGURE 2.7 Common lesions in the posterior aspect of the forearm. (**a**) Psoriatic plaque. (**b**) Rheumatoid nodules. (**c**) Gouty tophy (inspection could suggest olecranon bursitis but the lesion was firm on palpation)

Regional Clinical Examination

Observation

The first thing to look for is swelling around the elbow, which is common in cases of bursitis. The posterior aspect of the forearm and elbow is often the site of psoriatic plaques and rheumatoid nodules, which present as hard, painless subcutaneous lumps adhering to the deep planes. As a rule, there will be other signs of rheumatoid arthritis. There may also be gouty tophi, nodular accumulations of urate crystals with typical crepitus on compression. The clinical context will usually suggest gout (Fig. 2.7).

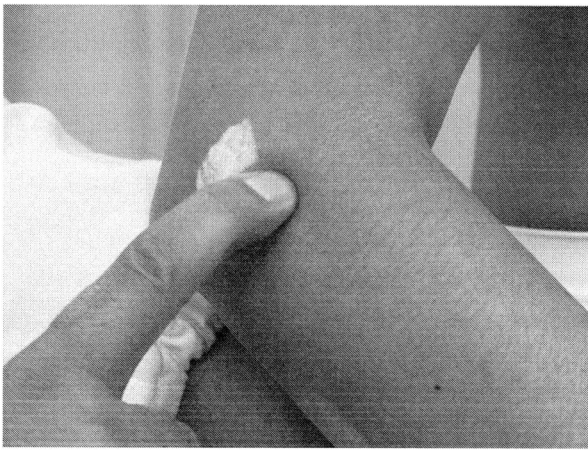

FIGURE 2.8 Palpating the insertion of the extensors of the wrist and hand, just below the lateral epicondyle

Joint synovitis and effusion may cause visible swelling or other signs of inflammation, but they are better identified by palpation.

Palpation

Palpation should focus on four main points:

1. Immediately below the lateral epicondyle, at the insertion of the common tendon insertion of the extensors of the wrist and fingers, the site of lateral epicondylitis (tennis elbow – Fig. 2.8)
2. Immediately below the medial epicondyle, in the common tendon of the flexors, the site of medial epicondylitis (golfer's elbow – Fig. 2.9)

In either case, the exact point of maximum pain varies and we should palpate the whole tendinous part from the posterior to the anterior face, exerting adequate pressure.

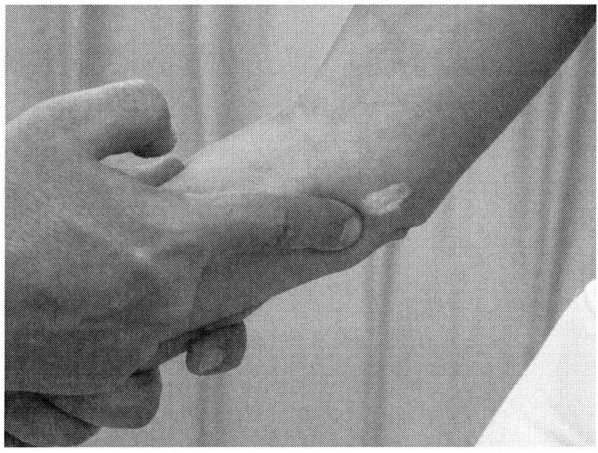

FIGURE 2.9 Palpating the insertion of the flexors of the wrist and hand, just below the medial epicondyle

3. The olecranon bursa and nodules should be palpated to ascertain their texture, tenderness, effusion or local warmth.
4. Palpation of the joint is not easy, as the anterior aspect is covered by muscle and there are no clear bone references on the posterior face. The examination for effusion or swelling is more effective if you insert the tips of your thumb and medial finger into the grooves on each side of the olecranon. The elbow is then fully flexed and extended (Fig. 2.10.). Any effusion or voluminous synovial swelling will be expelled by the olecranon in extension, as it occupies the olecranon fossa of the humerus. This is felt by the palpating fingers as a protrusion occurring with extension and disappearing with flexion of the elbow. There may be perceptible crepitus, if the cartilage is damaged.

Swelling and tenderness caused by synovitis may also be detected by palpating over the head of the radius. It is perceptible as a rounded bony structure on the posterolateral aspect of the elbow, below the epicondyle.

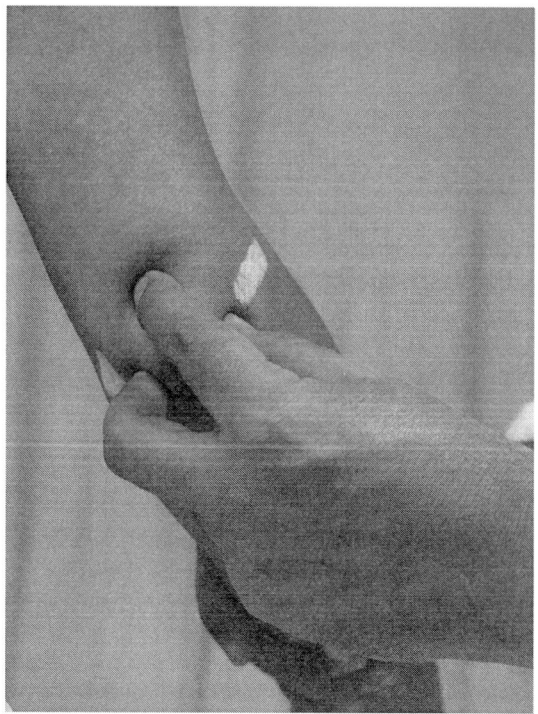

FIGURE 2.10 Examining for swelling or effusion of the elbow joints: during extension fingertips placed either side of the olecranon may sense the expulsion of excess joint fluid

Slide the back of your hand along the posterior and anterior face of the elbow to look for a local increase in temperature.

Mobilization

The normal elbow is capable of about 145° flexion. Extension goes as far as 0°, and there may be hyperextension of up to −10° in many normal women. More pronounced hyperextension may be part of a *hypermobility syndrome* and may be associated with pain caused by subluxation and distension of the ligaments.

Active and passive movements of the elbow are not affected in lateral or medial epicondylitis. Joint diseases frequently result in early joint limitation, particularly extension, which the patient may fail to mention and may not have noticed. Occasionally, there is noticeable crepitus. Limitation of passive supination and pronation points to disease of the proximal or (especially) distal radioulnar joints.

Pain in epicondylitis can be exacerbated by resisted extension of the wrist. The same is the case with flexion in medial epicondylitis (Fig. 2.11a and b).

If the local examination is normal, the possibility of referred pain from the wrist, shoulder or cervical spine should be considered. In these cases, pain is exacerbated by movements or palpation of these structures.

Neurological Examination

In cases of suspected nerve root lesion, we must conduct a local neurological examination. The elbow receives sensitive innervation from C5 and C6 on the radial aspect and from T1 on the ulnar side. Both should be examined for sensitivity to pin-prick and touch.

To assess muscle strength, test the following movements:

1. Resisted extension – triceps (radial nerve, C7)
2. Resisted flexion – biceps and brachialis (musculocutaneous nerve, C5/6)
3. Supination against resistance – biceps (musculocutaneous nerve, C5/6) and supinator (radial nerve, C6)
4. Pronation against resistance – pronator teres (median nerve, C6) and pronator quadratus (anterior interosseous branch, C8/T1)

Assess the reflexes of the biceps (musculocutaneous nerve, C5/6) and triceps (radial nerve, C7).

To test for ulnar nerve compression, suggested by paresthesia along the medial aspect of the forearm and hand, percuss over the ulnar tunnel (Tinel's test). If this reproduces the

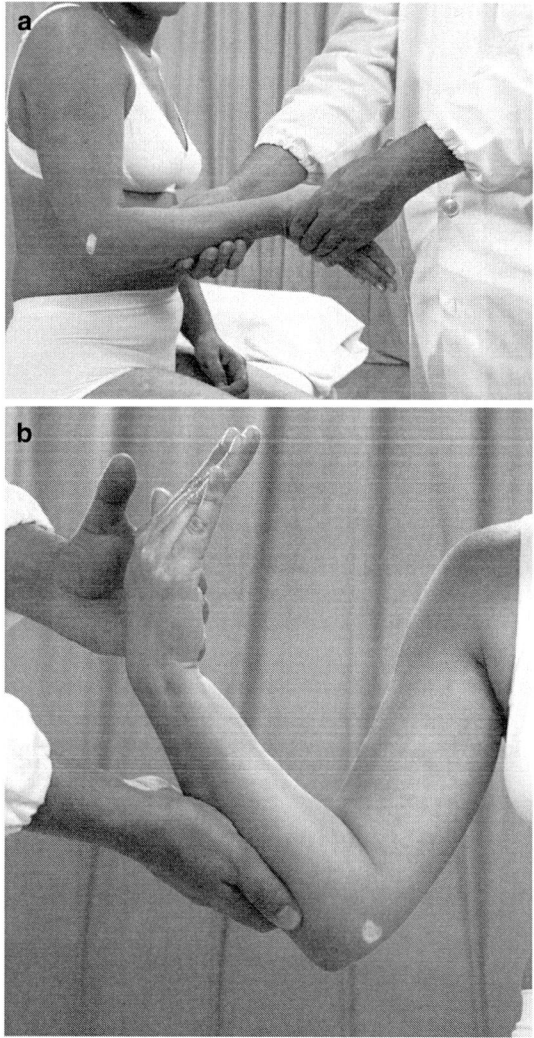

FIGURE 2.11 In lateral epicondylitis, the resisted extension of the wrist may induce pain in the lateral aspect of the elbow. (a) In medial epicondylitis, resisted flexion of the wrist will cause pain in the medial aspect of the elbow (b)

symptoms, ulnar nerve entrapment is likely, though false positives are common. Deep palpation or percussion of the exit points of the anterior and posterior interosseous nerves can trigger typical symptoms, suggesting nerve entrapment (pronator syndrome and radial tunnel syndrome, respectively).

Typical Cases
2.A. Elbow Pain (I)
Mário Alberto, a 38-year old computer operator, came to the surgery because of pain in his right elbow and forearm, which had started 3 months earlier and become progressively more intense and troublesome. The pain appeared only with movement and got worse when he picked up any objects, even light ones. When asked, he located the pain on the lateral aspect of the elbow and proximal forearm.

He denied any other joint problems, including his shoulder or cervical region. He had generally enjoyed good health until then.

The general rheumatologic examination revealed no pain or limited mobility. Active and passive movements of the elbow were easy and painless. There was no swelling, crepitus or local increase in temperature.

Was our clinical examination complete?

Compression of the common tendon of the extensors, below the epicondyle, caused intense pain, similar to the spontaneous pain and this was reproduced by resisted extension of the right wrist.

What is your diagnosis?
Would you require any tests?
What treatment would you suggest for this patient?

The observations above established a diagnosis of tennis elbow, with no need for additional tests. We suggested local application of a topical non-steroidal anti-inflammatory and a splint. We also recommended that he used supports for his forearms when working. Two weeks later, the patient had not improved. We gave him a local injection of 0.5 cc methylpred-nisolone (20 mg) around the tendon and recommended abso-lute rest of his right arm for 24 hours. We repeated our earlier suggestions in order to avoid any recurrences.

Please note: the symptoms of medial epicondylitis are much the same, but are located in the medial aspect of the elbow. Resisted flexion of the wrist exacerbates the pain. Work or leisure activities involving repeated forced flexion of the fingers (e.g. tennis, golf,… or an electoral campaign…) are predisposing factors. The treatment is very similar.

Lateral and Medial Epicondylitis
Main Points
These syndromes are very common in clinical practice, and are the most frequent causes of isolated pain in the elbow.

They appear most often in young and middle-aged adults, and are related to work or leisure activities requir-ing repeated flexion and extension of the wrists and fingers.

The pain has a mechanical rhythm and is located on the lateral aspect of the elbow and forearm in lateral epicon-dylitis and in the medial aspect in medial epicondylitis.

Active and passive mobility of the elbow is not affected.

Palpation of the corresponding muscle insertions causes intense pain.

Treatment is conservative: topical non-steroidal anti-inflammatories and splints or an elastic bandage in the ini-tial stages and corticosteroid injections in persistent cases.

Physical therapy may be important if the symptoms persist. Tendon decompression may be necessary in stubborn, incapacitating cases.

The patient should be advised about high-risk activities and ways of avoiding lesions such as suggesting palm-upwards method of lifting in lateral epicondylitis.

NB: Symptoms suggesting epicondylitis or medial epicondylitis may only be the most visible face of generalized pain or fibromyalgia. You must explore all the clinical symptoms.

Typical Cases
2.B. Elbow Pain (II)

José Silvares had been going to the same health centre for many years and suffered from tophaceous gouty arthritis that was resistant to treatment. He had had multiple episodes of migratory, recurring monoarthritis mainly affecting joints in his lower limbs. Over the years, he had developed progressive deformities in his hands and feet.

He went to emergency because of continuous, incapacitating pain in his left elbow. It had all started a few days earlier after a small local trauma which broke the skin and burst one of the nodules that he had had there for a long time. A whitish liquid came out, like liquid plaster. Inflammation had begun 2 days later…

On examination, we found that José had multiple nodules in his hands and elbows. The posterior aspect of his left elbow was very swollen and red, with fluctuation and pain on palpation. Attempts at mobilizing the joint caused intense local pain.

His family doctor decided to send him to hospital immediately because of suspected infection. The diagnosis of septic bursitis (*Staphylococcus aureus*) on top of tophaceous gout was confirmed. It required prolonged, systemic antibiotic treatment and local surgical debridement.

Olecranon Bursitis

Main Points

This is reflected by swelling and pain over the olecranon. Palpation shows the presence of a fluctuant mass confirming presence of fluid.

Chronic bursitis caused by repeated trauma may develop without pain or signs of inflammation.

Intense pain, redness and local warmth suggest septic or microcrystalline bursitis. Olecranon bursitis may represent local involvement by polyarthritis (e.g. rheumatoid arthritis), in which case the signs of inflammation are moderate and the clinical context is suggestive.

Acute bursitis requires urgent treatment and should be referred to a specialized clinic. In other cases, the treatment depends on the underlying condition.

Typical Cases

2.C. Elbow Pain (III)

The patient, a 42-year old woman, was followed up by us and her family doctor for typical rheumatoid arthritis: chronic, symmetrical, additive polyarthritis, involving the small joints in the hands, wrists, elbows and ankles. The disease was well controlled on stable doses of immunosuppressant treatment, with no significant signs of inflammatory activity for the previous 2 years. We observed the patient every 6 months and her family doctor saw her in between.

At one of these visits, she complained to her doctor of growing inflammatory pain in her right elbow, which she attributed to hard farm work. Her doctor suspected reactivation of the arthritis in this location and asked us to examine her as soon as possible.

What would you expect to find on examination?

We confirmed the diagnosis. Although the joint was normal on inspection, extension was reduced (with fixed flexion deformity of ~15°), and we were unable to increase the range with passive mobilization. Palpation of the peri-olecranon grooves during flexion/extension of the elbow showed swelling and slight pain. Palpation of the radial head was also painful. There was no obvious local warmth or redness over the elbow. Examination of the other joints revealed only moderate synovitis of a few MCP joints.

What tests and/or treatment would you recommend?

There were no signs or symptoms suggesting general reactivation of the rheumatoid arthritis. We aspirated synovial fluid, which showed a high neutrophil count (8500/mm³). Tests for crystals and bacteria were negative, thus excluding the possibility of septic arthritis. We decided to administer an intra-articular injection of a long-acting corticosteroid and asked the patient to keep her arm in a sling for 2 days. She was advised to do progressive exercises to recover the range of movement of the joint, following the period of rest.

We saw the patient two weeks later. The problem had resolved and she was back to normal.

Arthritis of the Elbow
Main Points
The elbow is often involved in polyarthritis, but is rarely the site of the initial episode. Monoarthritis of the elbow should suggest the possibility of septic or microcrystalline arthritis.

Osteoarthritis of the elbow is rare and suggests an underlying metabolic cause.

The following signs and symptoms point to arthritis:

- Inflammatory pain;
- Restricted motion and pain on active and passive mobilization;
- Swelling and pain on palpation of the joint;
- Redness and local warmth (inconsistent).

It is essential to conduct a systematic enquiry and general examination to look for symptoms and signs of a more general disease.

The treatment depends on the underlying condition.

The elbow is highly sensitive to the inflammatory process. Irreversible damage to the joint can appear in a very short time, with limitations of extension and supination/pronation. This justifies the early use of intra-articular treatment.

Monoarthritis of the elbow should be addressed in the same way as other monoarthritides.

Special Situations

Although they are relatively rare, two syndromes involving peripheral nerve entrapment can cause pain of the forearm and may not be detected in our suggested clinical examination.

Radial Tunnel Syndrome

This syndrome should be suspected when the patient describes deep, diffuse pain on the lateral and posterior aspect of the forearm. In some cases it may involve the lateral face of the elbow, suggesting lateral epicondylitis. The predominance of symptoms in the forearm, the presence of (inconsistent) paresthesia and muscle weakness favor this diagnosis.

The radial nerve may be compressed by abnormal fibrous bands behind the radial head. The posterior interosseous nerve, a branch of the radial nerve, is more often affected when it passes through the supinator muscle on the posterior aspect of the forearm, immediately below the elbow (about 30% of people have a fibrous arc here).

The following findings in the clinical exam are particularly suggestive:

- Reproduction of the pain by forced passive flexion or resisted extension of the middle finger
- Reproduction of the pain by extreme pronation of the forearm with flexion of the wrist
- Pain when pressure is applied with a tourniquet or sphyg-momanometer cuff on the proximal forearm
- Weakness of extension of the little finger (posterior interosseous nerve)
- Pain on deep palpation of the posterolateral face of the forearm about 5 cm below the epicondyle (Fig. 2.4)
- Positive Tinel's sign at this site (posterior interosseous nerve) or over the radial head (radial nerve)[2]

The electromyogram/nerve conduction study is normal, except in very advanced phases of nerve lesion.

The treatment involves rest and mild exercise to begin with, then local anesthetic and corticosteroid injections if the symptoms persist. The use of splints or elastic bandages may bring relief, but the results vary. Surgical decompression may be necessary.

Pronator Syndrome

The anterior interosseous nerve, a branch of the median nerve, is compressed by the pronator teres muscle, 5–7 cm below the elbow.

---

[2]Tinel's (or Hoffman-Tinel's) sign consists of percussion on the site of potential compression of a nerve, preferably with a reflex hammer. The sign is positive if it causes tingling or pain in the innervation area.

This condition causes deep, undefined pain in the anterior aspect of the forearm. It tends to be continuous, although it is exacerbated by the use of the hands and wrists. Paresthesia in the area of the median nerve is suggestive but unfortunately inconsistent.

Evidence of muscular weakness or reproduction of the pain on resisted pronation suggests this diagnosis. In severe, chronic cases, there may be hypesthesia in the median nerve area. Deep compression of the site for about 30 seconds reproduces or exacerbates the symptoms (Fig. 2.3). The tourniquet test described above may also be positive.

The treatment is similar to that indicated for radial tunnel syndrome.

Please note: In either situation, do not forget to explore the possibility of generalized pain or fibromyalgia.

Diagnostic Tests

Generally speaking, diagnostic tests are unproductive and rarely necessary in regional pain of the elbow. Signs of joint disease or a history of trauma justify standard x-rays.

The presence of arthritis or acute bursitis of unexplained origin warrants fluid aspiration and analysis to look for crystals and bacteria and determine the total cell count and predominant cell type. Arthrocentesis of the elbow requires technical experience and laboratory facilities for synovial fluid studies. Suspected nerve entrapment may warrant electromyographic/nerve conduction studies.

Treatment

The treatment of the most common causes of pain in the elbow and forearm has already been described and is within the scope of general practitioners. Avoid administering local injections if you are not trained or experienced in this technique.

When Should the Patient be Referred to a Specialist?
Clinical signs and/or imaging results indicating mechanical or inflammatory joint disease of unknown cause.[3] In the case of arthritis, the referral should be urgent.

Clinically significant tendonitis or bursitis that is resistant to the measures used in general practice.

Persistent, debilitating pain of unknown origin.

---

[3]Osteoarthritis of the elbow is very rare. If there is no relevant history of trauma or previous arthritis, it almost always signifies metabolic joint disease, which requires appropriate etiologic investigation.

Chapter 3
Regional Syndromes
The Wrist and Hand

The wrist and hand are extremely valuable sources of medical information. They are often the site of regional pathologies. Even more important, however, the hands provide significant and often diagnostic evidence in a variety of systemic rheumatic diseases. For these reasons, it is essential to master the clinical examination of this area. "*The hand is the rheumatology patient's calling card.*"

Functional Anatomy

The wrist and the hand make up a complex structural unit. While it is not essential for the clinician to master all the details of the anatomy, it is important to understand some basic aspects.

The wrist is made up of several joints (Fig. 3.1):

1. The radiocarpal joint, which is used for flexion/extension and adduction/abduction;
2. The distal radioulnar joint, which is involved in the supination and pronation of the forearm;
3. The intercarpal and carpo-metacarpal joints, which are involved in wrist movements, especially during forced flexion. The synovial cavity of the distal radioulnar joint is independent of the radiocarpal joint. All the others interconnect (except for the first carpometacarpal joint).

J.A.P. da Silva, A.D. Woolf, *Rheumatology of the Upper Limbs in Clinical Practice*, DOI 10.1007/978-1-4471-2242-5_3,
© Springer-Verlag London Limited 2012

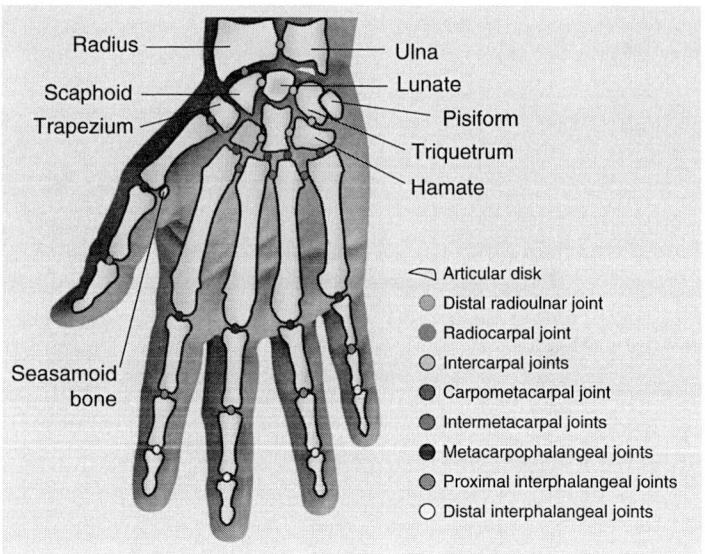

Radius — Ulna
Scaphoid — Lunate
Trapezium — Pisiform
Triquetrum
Hamate

◁ Articular disk
● Distal radioulnar joint
● Radiocarpal joint
○ Intercarpal joints
● Carpometacarpal joint
● Intermetacarpal joints
● Metacarpophalangeal joints
● Proximal interphalangeal joints
○ Distal interphalangeal joints

Seasamoid
bone

FIGURE 3.1 Bones and joints of the hand and wrist

The carpus consists of eight bones arranged in two transverse rows. These bones have many articulations between them and are stabilized by intrinsic ligaments.

The carpus articulates proximally, via the radiocarpal joint, with the distal extremity of the radius laterally, and medially with an articular disc (the triangular ligament of the carpus), which separates the radius from the distal extremity of the ulna.

The bones in the second row of the carpus articulate with the proximal extremities of the metacarpals. The joints that surround the base of the second and third metacarpals are practically immobile and, although they can be the site of pathology (e.g. in rheumatoid arthritis), they are not amenable to individual clinical examination. The fourth and fifth carpometacarpal joints provide the adjacent metacarpals with a slight capacity for flexion. In most people, the radiocarpal, intercarpal and carpometacarpal joints (second to fifth) are connected by a common synovial cavity. This explains their combined involvement in arthritis when the wrist is affected.

The first carpometacarpal joint, which joins the trapezium to the base of the first metacarpal (first carpometacarpal joint or trapeziometacarpal joint), is particularly important. It has an independent capsule and synovial cavity. It is highly mobile (flexion/extension and adduction/abduction) and plays an extremely important role in the global function of the human hand, by allowing opposition of the thumb and fingers. It is often the site of osteoarthritis and deserves special attention during clinical examination of the hand.

The five metacarpophalangeal (MCP) joints are independent and are responsible essentially for flexion (about 90°) and extension (up to −10°), with slight adduction and abduction. The mobility of the first metacarpophalangeal joint (MCP1, of the thumb), with two sesamoid bones on the palmar face, is much more limited, not exceeding 30° flexion. The morphology of the proximal interphalangeal joints (PIPs) is similar to that of the metacarpophalangeals, permitting only flexion (90–100°) with 0° extension. The range of extension of the thumb interphalangeal joint (IFP1) is greater (45–60°), while flexion is more limited (80–90°).

There are four distal interphalangeal joints (DIPs, from the index to the little finger), with flexion of up to 90° and extension from 0 to −10°.

In normal circumstances, the segments of each finger are aligned along the same axis, in a slightly radial arrangement in relation to the axis of the wrist when at rest. In complete, forced flexion, the fingertips touch each other and press firmly into the palm.

Mobilization of the wrists and fingers depends on a large number of muscles joining the humerus and bones of the forearm to the fingers. Functionally, we can divide them into three groups. The flexors of the fingers are located along the palm face of the wrist and hand and the extensors along the dorsal face. The tendons of the long abductor and short extensor of the thumb run along the lateral aspect of the wrist.

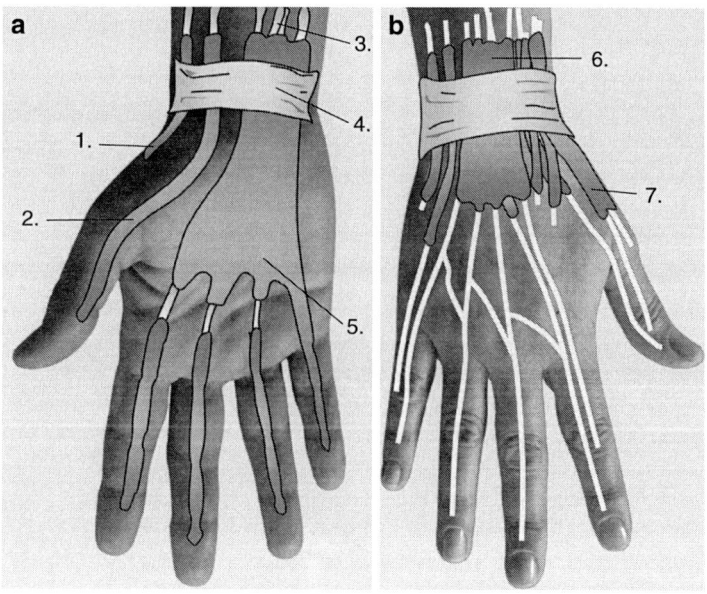

FIGURE 3.2 Tendon sheaths of the hand and wrist flexors. (**a**) Flexor tendons. 1. Flexor carpi radialis. 2. Flexor pollicis longus. 3. Flexor digitorum superficialis and profundus. 4. Flexor retinaculum. 5. Common sheath of flexor muscles. (**b**) Tendon sheaths of the hand and wrist extensors. Common variant. 6. Extensor digitorum and extensor indicis. 7. Tendon sheath of abductor pollicis longus and extensor pollicis brevis muscles

These muscles insert in the phalanges by means of long tendons surrounded by synovial sheaths. As these structures often participate in the inflammatory processes, it is important to pay them particular attention. On the palm face, the tendon of the long flexor of the thumb on the radial side is covered by an independent sheath that extends from the distal forearm to the first interphalangeal joint. In most people, the other flexors are covered by a common tendon sheath that extends as far as the distal interphalangeal joint of the little finger, ending in the palm over the other tendons. The flexors of the index, middle and ring finger have independent synovial sheaths extending from the palm to the distal interphalangeal joint (Fig. 3.2). The

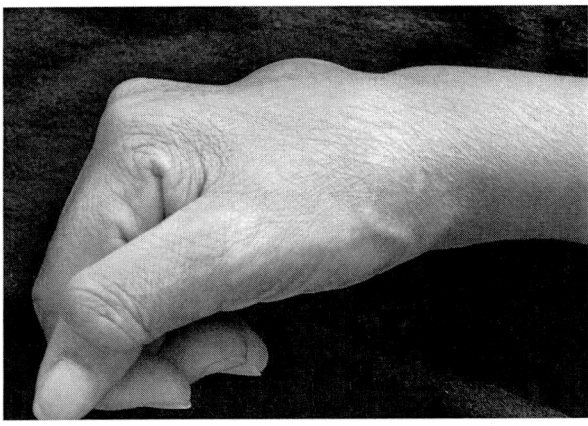

FIGURE 3.3 Tenosynovitis of the extensor tendons at the wrist may present as an hour-glass shaped swelling, due to the effect of the extensor retinaculum of the wrist

tendon sheaths do not communicate with the cavity of the underlying joints.

The sheaths of the extensors are more numerous (usually six) and variable (Fig. 3.2a). It is worth remembering the one that envelops the tendons of the long abductor and short extensor of the thumb. It runs along the lateral aspect of the wrist, constituting the anterior border of the anatomical snuffbox. Inflammation of this synovial sheath is called DeQuervain's tenosynovitis. The extensor retinaculum of the carpus forms a fibrous band over these synovial sheaths and cinches them, so that tenosynovitis of the extensors is frequently reflected by an hour-glass shaped swelling (Fig. 3.3).

Arranged between the metacarpals are the intrinsic muscles of the hand (the interosseous and lumbrical muscles), which reinforce the flexion of the metacarpophalangeal joints. Atrophy of these muscles is common in cases of chronic arthritis and neuropathic lesions, and is clinically detectable.

The hand is innervated by the radial, median and ulnar nerves. The radial nerve innervates the extensor muscles of

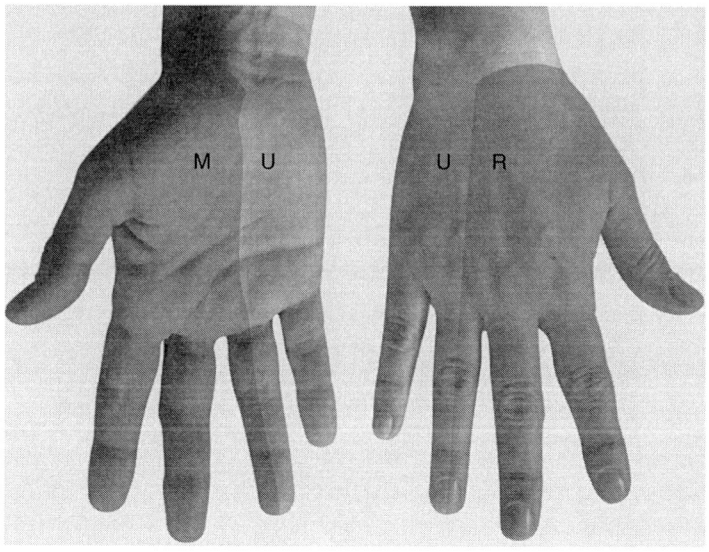

FIGURE 3.4 Sensory inervation of the hand. **M.** Median nerve. **U.** Ulnar nerve. **R.** Radial nerve

the wrist and fingers and is responsible for the sensitivity in the lateral half of the dorsal aspect of the hand and most of the dorsal face of the thumb, and index and middle fingers (Fig. 3.4). The median and ulnar nerves innervate the flexor muscles of the wrist and fingers. The median nerve provides sensations for the palmar aspect of the thumb to the middle finger and the external half of the ring finger, together with the corresponding area of the palm. The area of sensation provided by the ulnar nerve includes the little finger, the medial half of the ring finger and the corresponding ulnar part of the hand, on the palmar and dorsal faces. It should be remembered, however, that there is considerable variation in these cutaneous distributions.

The median nerve reaches the hand through the carpal tunnel, a non-distensible osteotendinous structure formed posteriorly by the bones and joints of the wrist and their capsule, in a concave form, and limited anteriorly by the flexor

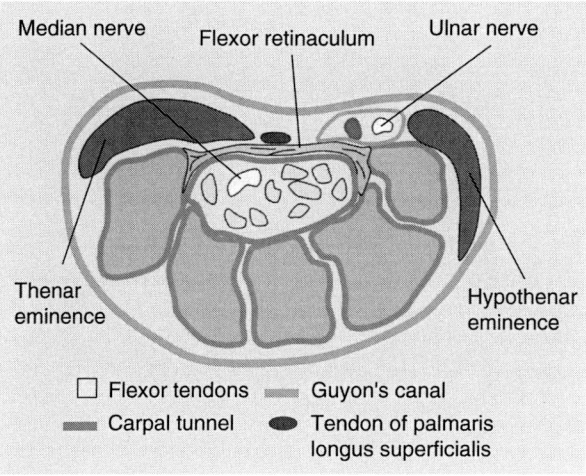

FIGURE 3.5 Carpal tunnel and ulnar tunnel (Guyon's canal)

retinaculum. This channel houses all the flexor tendons and their sheaths, together with the median nerve, arteries and veins (Fig. 3.5). Understandably, inflammation in the synovium of the joints or tendon sheaths, fibrous alterations, bony deformities or fluid retention in this area can result in compression and subsequent dysfunction of the median nerve. This causes carpal tunnel syndrome. The ulnar nerve runs anteriorly to the retinaculum, and externally to the pisiform in its own canal (Guyon's canal) where it can also be compressed.

Radiological Anatomy

In x-rays of the wrists and hands (Fig. 3.6) examine all the joints from the wrist to the DIPs, running along each articular row. Note the size and regularity of the articular spaces and the presence of periarticular osteopenia or subchondral sclerosis. Examine any swelling or calcification of the soft tissue. If in doubt, compare with the other side.

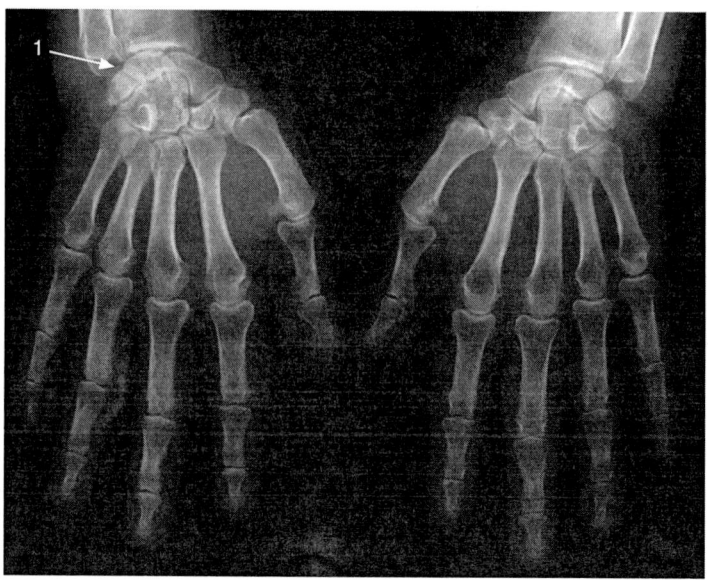

FIGURE 3.6 Normal radiography of the wrists and hand – antero-posterior view. 1. Area of projection of the triangular ligament of the carpus

In normal circumstances, the borders of the bones inside and on the periphery of the joints are regular, with a well-defined cortex. Note any calcification in the triangular ligament of the carpus and at the edge of the joints. Look for erosions (particularly of the styloid process of the ulna, MCPs and PIPs) and osteophytes (mainly in the first CMC, PIPs and DIPs). An oblique angle (Fig. 3.7) sometimes reveals erosions or osteophytes that are not detectable in an anteroposterior view.

Common Causes of Pain in the Wrist and Hand

The hand and wrist are common sites of pain, either limited to the region or as part of generalized rheumatic diseases (Table 3.1).

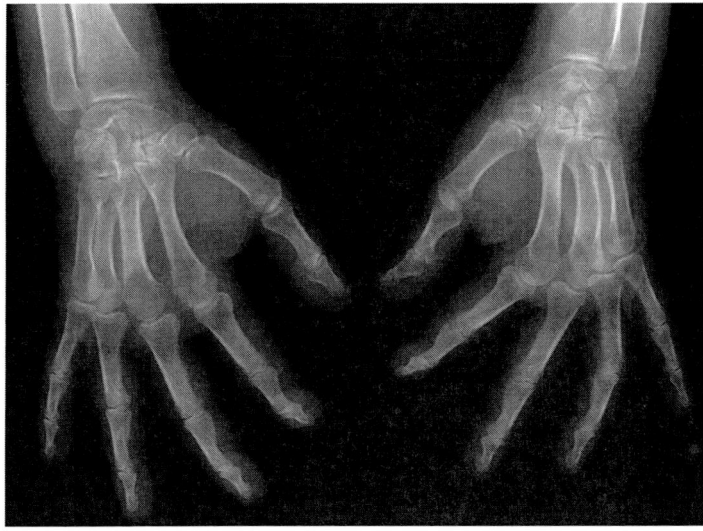

FIGURE 3.7 Normal radiography of the hand and wrist – oblique view

Overall, carpal tunnel syndrome is the most common condition. De Quervain's tenosynovitis and osteoarthritis of the trapezo-metacarpal joint are also often found.

Both osteoarthritis and the different types of inflammatory arthritis frequently involve the hands, and the distribution of affected hand joints may be highly informative for reaching a correct diagnosis.

The Enquiry

A clinical enquiry with a patient whose complaints predominate in the wrists and hands will naturally aim to establish the clinical characteristics of each of the conditions mentioned above, with special attention to the aspects that distinguish them from each other.

TABLE 3.1 Most common causes of pain in the wrist and hand

Structure	Lession	Clinical clues
	Carpal tunnel syndrome	Paresthesia of the hand confined to the area of the median nerve
		Predominantly at night and in the morning Tinel's and Phalen's signs
Peripheral nerves	Ulnar nerve syndrome	Paresthesia of the ulnar aspect of the forearm and hand.
		Tinel's sign of the ulnar tunnel in the elbow
	De Quervain's tenosynovitis	Pain in the lateral aspect of the wrist and thumb
		Mechanical rhythm
		Local pain on palpation
		Finkelstein's maneuver
Tendon sheaths and fascia	Tenosynovitis of the flexor tendons	Inflammatory or mechanical pain
		Limited active flexion of the fingers
		"Snapping" movement of the finger (trigger finger)
	Dupuytren's contracture	Fibrosis and contraction of the palmar fascia in the palmar aspect of the 3rd, 4th or 5th finger
	Osteoarthritis of the 1st carpometacarpal joint	Mechanical pain at the base of the thumb and radial aspect of the wrist
Joints	Nodal osteoarthritis	Mixed rhythm pain
		Proximal and distal interphalangeal joints
		Firm articular nodes
	Arthritis	Inflammatory pain
		Rubbery articular swelling
Referred	Cervical spine	Normal local examination
		Associated manifestations

It is important to take into account the relative prevalence of these different affections in general practice. Carpal tunnel syndrome, De Quervain's tenosynovitis, osteoarthritis of the 1st CMC and nodal osteoarthritis are much more common than inflammatory forms of arthritis. A thorough examination of the hands is mandatory in all patients, as it gives us a wealth of precise information that will help to narrow the differential diagnosis.

In this chapter we review the most important questions, assuming that the complaints are limited to the hands. However, a comprehensive, systemic enquiry is particularly important here, given that manifestations in the hands are frequently a sign of more disseminated diseases.

Where Exactly Does It Hurt?

In many cases, the patient indicates a reasonably precise area of pain, thus helping the doctor. As a rule, the pain due to osteoarthritis of the 1st CMC joint is limited to the base of the thumb and radial aspect of the wrist. The pain in De Quervain's tenosynovitis involves the same area, but may extend proximally to the forearm. In cases of mono- or oligoarthritis, the patient is usually able to identify the painful joints, which are often visibly swollen.

Patients sometimes say that the pain affects the "joints" of their hands. If several joints hurt, they will often say that they all hurt. We should not accept this at face value. It is hardly ever true! Ask the patient to place his hands on the desk and show you exactly which joints (or groups of joints) have been painful.

The exact distribution of the affected joints in the hand is invaluable in diagnosing a variety of joint diseases.

If the patient points to the palmar aspect of his hand or fingers, consider the possibility of tenosynovitis of the flexors, carpal tunnel syndrome or Dupuytren's contracture (the last of these is usually obvious on inspection and is usually painless). Many patients with carpal tunnel syndrome say that the pain or paresthesia affects the whole surface of the palm and not just the territory of the median nerve. Conversely, in ulnar nerve syndrome, the patient usually points to the ulnar border of the hand.

Patients with arthritis or osteoarthritis generally locate the pain on the dorsal face of the hand and fingers. Some patients describe typical trigger finger: one or more fingers hurt on flexion. If they are forcibly flexed, they "get stuck," and then spring free with a "snatching" or "triggering" movement when extended. Mobility is reasonable free, if forced flexion is avoided. This curious finding is diagnostic of stenosing tenosynovitis of the flexor tendons.

The patient very often has difficulty in pinpointing an exact location. The enquiry leaves an idea of imprecise, diffuse pain affecting most of the hand. This is an important clue to neurogenic or referred pain, which is extremely common in clinical practice. It is our cue to start asking more precise questions...

Is There Any Paresthesia?

What we need to find out is whether the pain is paresthetic in nature: "*Do you feel pins and needles in your hand? Does it go numb?*" If the answer is yes or even ambiguous, this reinforces the suspicion of neurogenic pain caused by cervical root compression or, more often, a peripheral nerve lesion. The rhythm of the pain is a strong characteristic of this syndrome.

Rhythm of the Pain

"*Does your pain have a special timing? Is it worse in the morning, later in the day, at night, only with movement?...*"

In carpal tunnel syndrome the answer is usually clear cut. The discomfort occurs most at night and early in the morning and gets better with the use of the hands. Note that this is an inflammatory rhythm! It might suggest arthritis, but then pain would be focused in the joints and is not dysesthetic.

The pain in osteoarthritis of the 1st CMC joint and De Quervain's tenosynovitis is usually related to manual work and disappears at rest.

Arthritis of the hand is usually accompanied by typical inflammatory pain. Patients may be more precise about morning stiffness affecting the hands than any other area.

How Did the Problem Begin?

The onset of arthritis and tenosynovitis is usually much faster (from hours to weeks) than osteoarthritis or nerve entrapment (from weeks to months).

Have There Been Any Signs of Inflammation?

Patients often describe swelling of the hands and this can be misleading. Ask about its location and daily rhythm.

In most cases of joint disease, the swelling is not diffuse but localized around one or more joints. If there is synovitis of the interphalangeal joints, the swelling is usually fusiform as the inflamed synovium is limited by the capsule. Patients with swelling of the metacarpophalangeal joints usually point to the knuckles.

Many patients will mention diffuse edema all over the hand or on all the fingers, however. If you cannot see the edema, this symptom is difficult to interpret. In many cases, the patient will find that this edema fluctuates with the menstrual cycle, which suggests premenstrual fluid retention. The sensation of morning swelling of the hands is also common in patients with carpal tunnel syndrome, even without any clinical evidence.

Patients with fibromyalgia often mention diffuse and generally "accentuated" swelling in their hands. A variety of factors may contribute to the prevalence of this symptom in these patients, although it is not particularly important. It may be misleading, however, leading the physician to consider a variety of possibilities if the highly variable symptoms of fibromyalgia are not taken into account.

A description of redness, if consistent, deserves attention, as it is not found in many situations: infection, microcrystalline arthritis and psoriatic arthritis. It is rare in rheumatoid arthritis and very rare in osteoarthritis.

Ask the patient whether the color of his hands changes when they are exposed to cold. If it does, especially in three phases (pale → cynanotic → red), this indicates Raynaud's phenomenon, which is always significant. Note that this phenomenon is often accompanied by paresthesia and pain, which may be the only cause for complaint.

Occasionally a patient says that a whole finger is red, swollen and painful. This can usually be verified by examination. If the examination confirms the presence of "dactylitis," this lends more weight to the possibility of infection, sarcoidosis or psoriatic arthritis.

The General Enquiry

It is always important to find out whether there is pain in any other locations. This is particularly important when the enquiry suggests arthropathy of the wrist or hand joints. For example, associated inflammatory back pain would suggest the possibility of seronegative spondylarthropathy The symmetrical involvement of proximal metacarpophalangeal and interphalangeal joints indicates rheumatoid arthritis and other connective tissue diseases. Cervical pain or pain in the forearm may indicate referred pain.

The patient's general state of health and associated diseases are also important. A recent myocardial infarction may be responsible for Dressler's syndrome. Hypothyroidism can cause carpal tunnel syndrome. Raynaud's phenomenon is a clue to disease of the connective tissue, vasculitis or nerve compression upstream. Chronic obstructive pulmonary disease and lung cancer may account for clubbed fingers. Hepatitis or rubella infection may be the cause of reactive polyarthritis. Diabetes mellitus can have quite curious effects on the hands...

The presence of other manifestations, outside the hands, may lead you to consider a different "main syndrome."

Regional Examination

The clinical examination of the wrist and hand is extraordinarily informative about a wide variety of rheumatic diseases. Because it is easy to do, it should always be complete and thorough in all patients with local symptoms, regardless of the diagnosis you suspect after the initial enquiry. You will often be surprised...

Observation

The palmar and dorsal aspects of the hand and wrist should be inspected carefully.

Examine the Skin

You may find signs here of such different diseases as psoriasis, systemic lupus erythematosus, scleroderma, dermatomyositis and vasculitis, among many others (Fig. 3.8). In cases of lupus, you occasionally find erythematous lesions on the dorsal aspect of the fingers, between the joints (Fig. 3.8a).

Reddish papules on the dorsal aspect of the finger joints (Gottron's papules) (Fig. 3.8b) are quite typical of dermatomyositis. They are sometimes associated with scaly erythematous lesions around the nails and ragged cuticles.

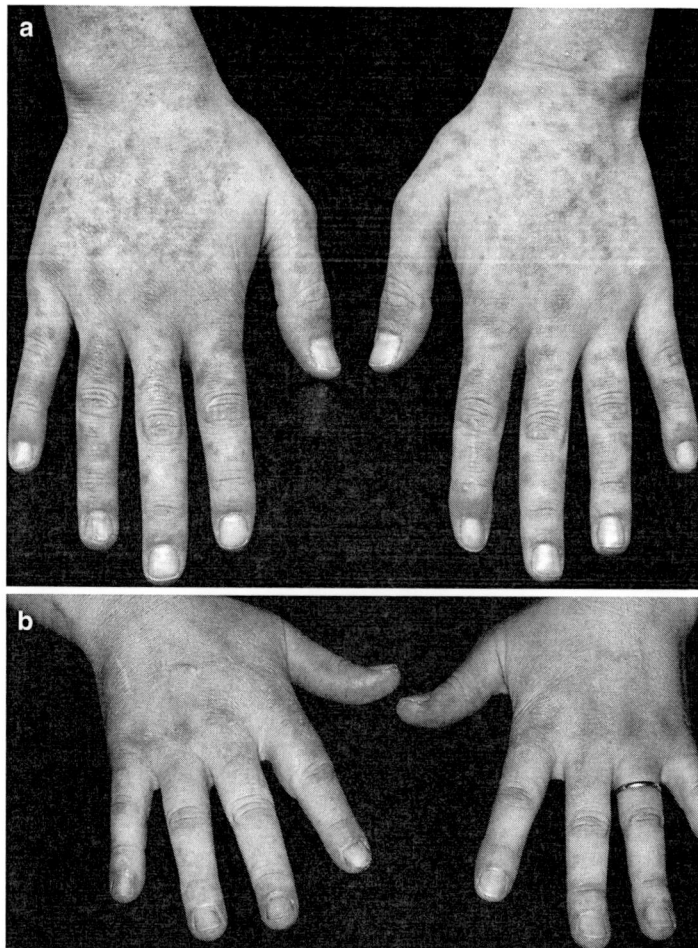

FIGURE 3.8 Hand skin changes in different rheumatic conditions. (a) Systemic lupus erythematosus. (b) Dermatomyositis. (c) Systemic sclerosis. (d) Subcutaneous infarcts

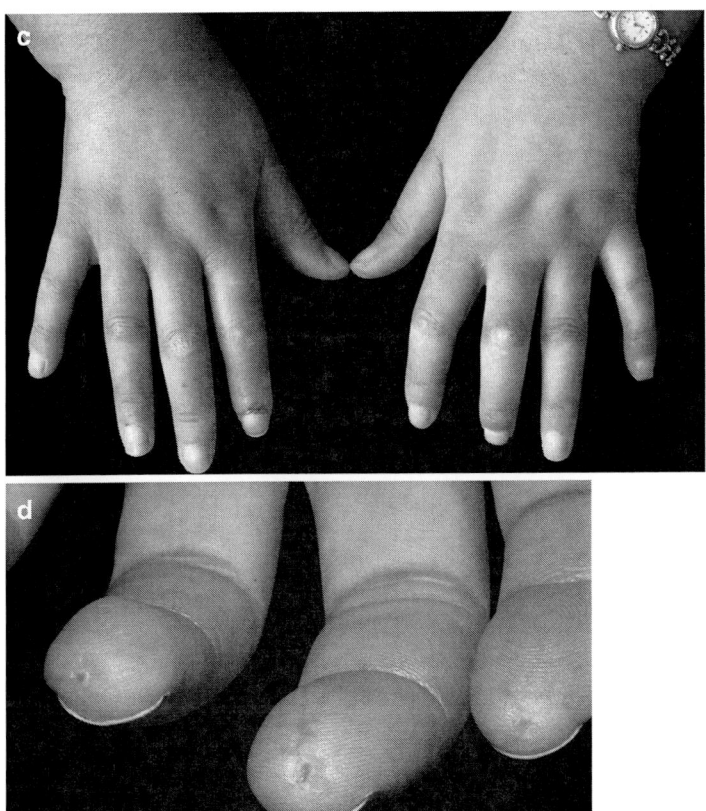

FIGURE 3.8 (continued)

Stretched, wax-like skin on the fingers is a strong indication of scleroderma, which is typical of progressive systemic sclerosis (Fig. 3.8c). The skin is hard and inflexible on palpation.

In patients with connective tissue diseases (especially lupus and systemic sclerosis) the pads of the fingers may be affected by calcinosis, ulceration and focal necrosis, making their surface irregular and atrophic (Fig. 3.8d). Dark point-like lesions at the edge of the nails may correspond to micro-infarctions indicating small vessel vasculitis, which is relatively common in these patients.

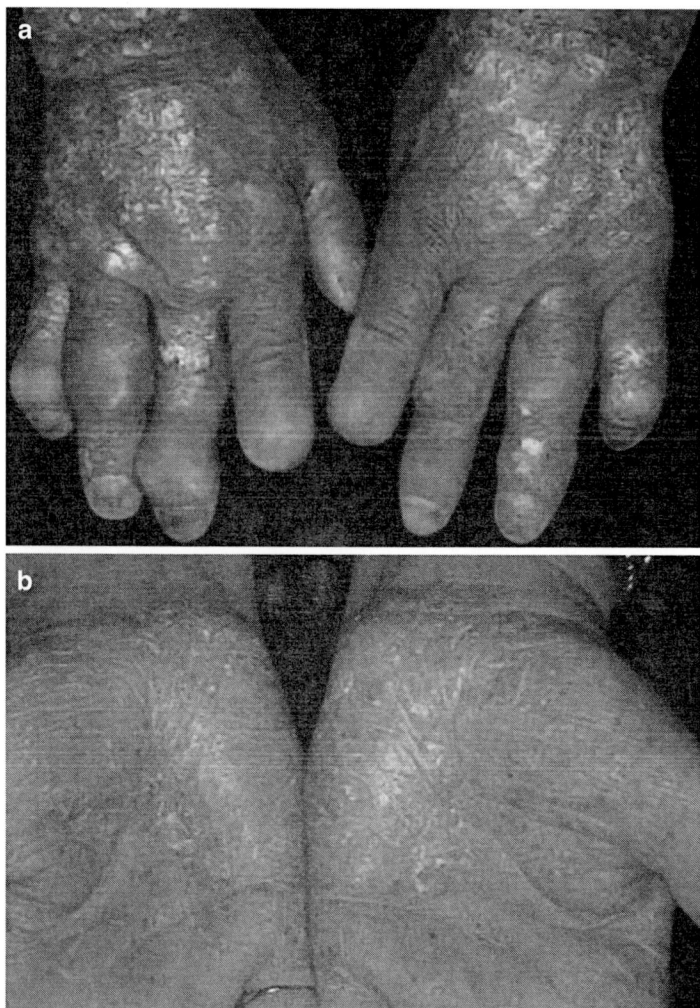

FIGURE 3.9 Psoriasis may present with typical patches in the hands (**a**) or palmar keratosis (**b**) Nail dystrophy and pitting (**c**) are more common when the distal interphalangeal joints are involved

FIGURE 3.9 (continued)

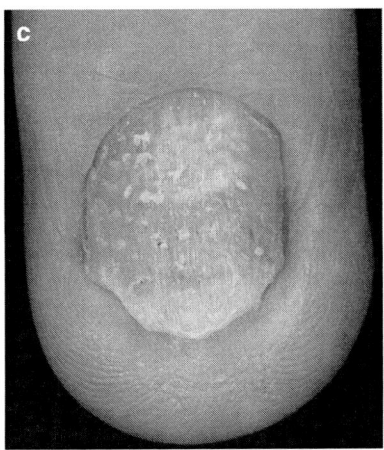

Be sure to look at the nails. Mycotic infections are common, but the presence of coarse nail dystrophy or pitting (Fig. 3.9) may be the only manifestation of psoriasis.[1]

Long-lasting corticosteroid therapy can cause skin atrophy, making it friable and prone to bruising. This is often prominent on the dorsal aspect of the hands.

Look for Signs of Muscle Atrophy

When carpal tunnel syndrome is chronic and severe it leads to atrophy of the muscles in the thenar eminence. Chronic lesions of the ulnar nerve lead to atrophy of the hypothenar eminence. Chronic arthritis of the wrist and hands often results in generalized atrophy of the intrinsic muscles of the hands, forming depressions between the tendons of the extensors (Fig. 3.10).

---

[1]Pitting consists in the presence of pointlike depressions in the ungual bed. Some authors consider that a total of 50 or more of these depressions in the ten nails of the hands confirms a diagnosis of psoriasis, even if there are no skin lesions.

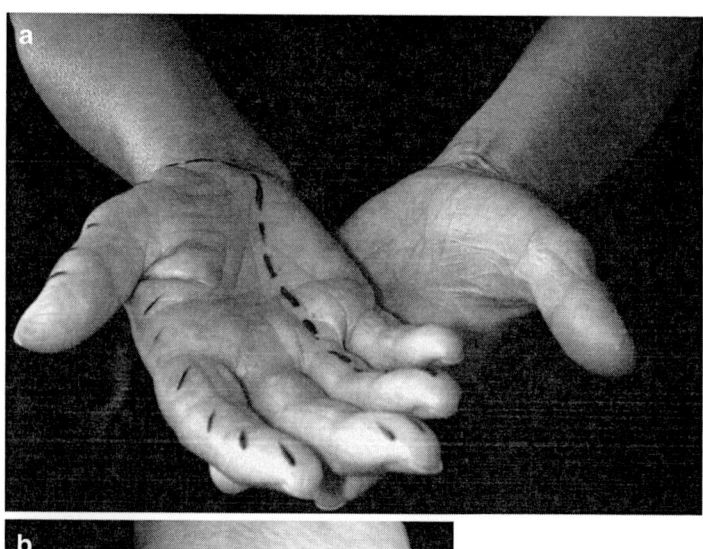

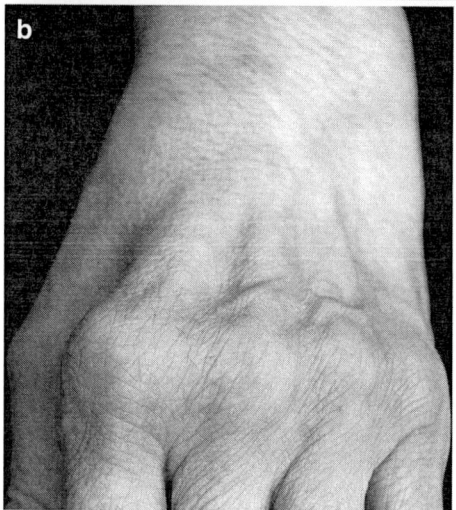

FIGURE 3.10 Muscle wasting in the hands. (**a**) Thenar eminence wasting is typical of advanced carpal tunnel syndrome. (**b**) Diffuse muscle wasting in chronic inflammatory polyarthritis

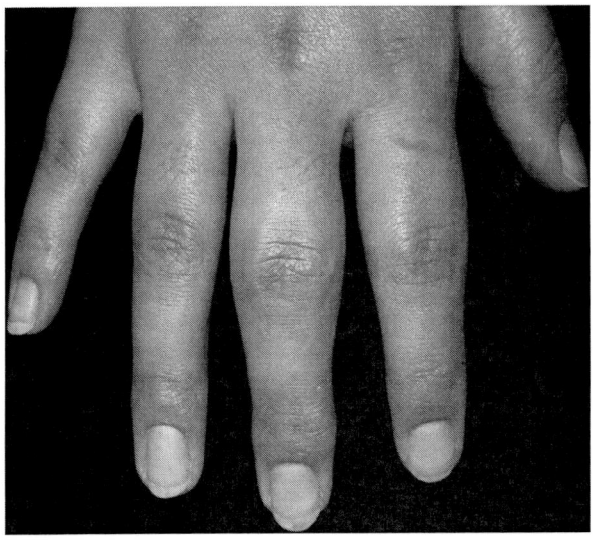

FIGURE 3.11 Fusiform swelling around the 2nd and 3rd proximal interphalangeal joints

Swelling

Visible swelling of the back of the wrist is usually due to tenosynovitis of the extensors. Bound by the posterior ligament of the carpus, these swollen structures assume the shape of an hourglass (Fig. 3.3).

Synovitis of the metacarpophalangeal joints may cause the recesses between the nodes of the fingers to fill up (Fig. 3.10). However, swelling of these joints should always be confirmed by palpation. The same is the case for the fusiform swelling around proximal interphalangeal joints – they are strongly suggestive of arthritis but it is palpation that will confirm the suspicion (Fig. 3.11).

Synovial cysts in the wrist (extensions of the synovium of the wrist due to partial rupture of the capsule), also known as ganglia, are common and usually painless. They present as a soft, localized swelling (Fig. 3.12).

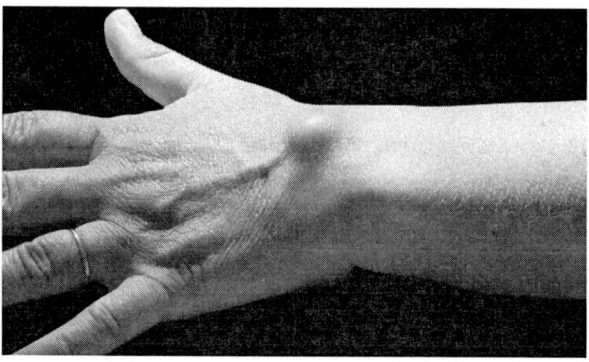

FIGURE 3.12 Synovial cyst of the wrist. The swelling is soft on palpation

Nodes

Nodes are relatively frequent in the hands. Rheumatoid nodules are usually found over the extension surface of the joints, and other areas subjected to friction. They are firm and painless, with no signs of inflammation, and adhere to the deep fascial planes (Fig. 3.13a).

Gouty tophi may form coarse swellings around the joints, if hyperuricaemia is not properly controlled. The superficial accumulation of urate crystals can give a suggestive whitish color (Fig. 3.14b). Firm palpation may elicit a typical crepitus.

Localized bony swellings on or near the dorsal aspect of the proximal (Bouchard's nodes) or distal (Heberden's nodes – Fig. 3.14) interphalangeal joints are highly suggestive of nodal osteoarthritis. This feature is quite different from the diffuse, spindle-shaped swelling observed in synovitis (Fig. 3.11).

Malalignment

Malalignment between the axis of adjacent bone segments is a sign of advanced joint disease. It is very common in the late stages of both rheumatoid arthritis and nodal osteoarthritis.

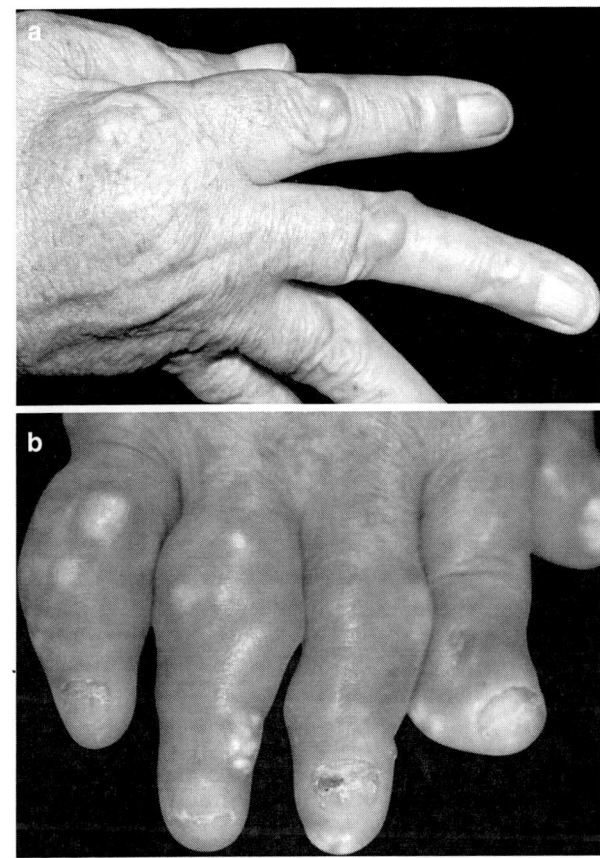

FIGURE 3.13 Nodules of the hands. (**a**) Rheumatoid nodules –
usually small with a regular surface. (**b**) Irregular nodules with white
deposits – gouty tophy

The typical deformities of these diseases are, however, quite
different.

In rheumatoid arthritis, malalignment occurs mainly along
the anteroposterior plane, as shown in Fig. 3.15a. The most
frequent deformities are in flexion or extension of the MCP,
PIP or DIP joints. Ulnar deviation of the fingers is common,
but the deviation takes place at the MCP joint. In advanced

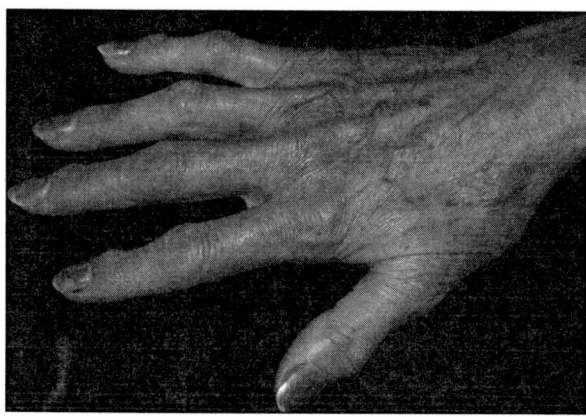

FIGURE 3.14 Nodal osteoarthritis of the hands. Discrete bony nodules around PIP (Bouchard nodes) and DIP joints (Heberden nodes)

nodal osteoarthritis, the hand may look disorganized and angular. There may be radial or ulnar deviation of one phalange over the other, which is accentuated by the nodules (Fig. 3.15b). An angular deformation at the base of the thumb suggests advanced osteoarthritis of the 1st CMC joint (Fig. 3.16).

The wrist is often deformed in arthritis. Synovial swelling is only visible when the disease is very active. In more advanced stages, however, the structural disorganization of the radiocarpal joint often leads to palmar subluxation of the carpus, making it look like the "back of a fork" (caput ulnae – Fig. 3.17).

Mobilization

First ask the patient to completely flex and extend his wrists. Then ask him to close his hand tight and slowly stretch his fingers as far as possible. If the active movement is limited, check whether passive mobilization is more complete.

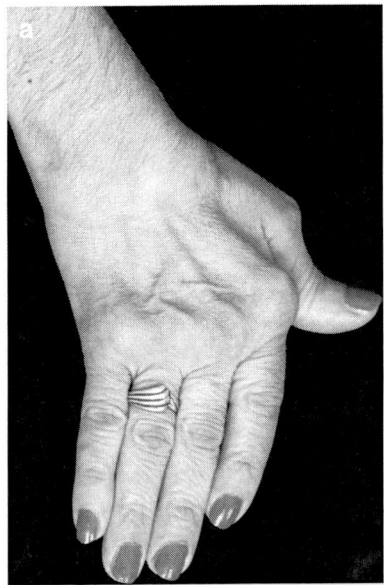

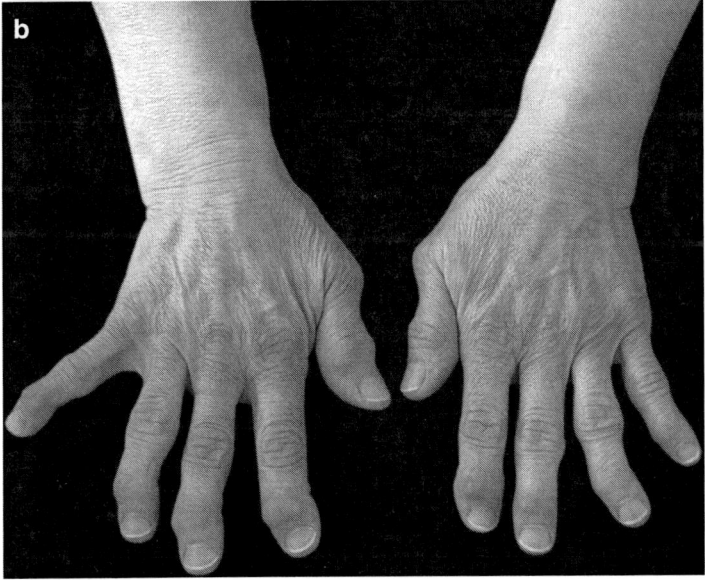

FIGURE 3.15 Finger deformity. (**a**) Ulnar deviation of the fingers in rheumatoid arthritis. (**b**) Nodular deformity of the finger, with deviations of one phalanx over the other in nodal osteoarthritis

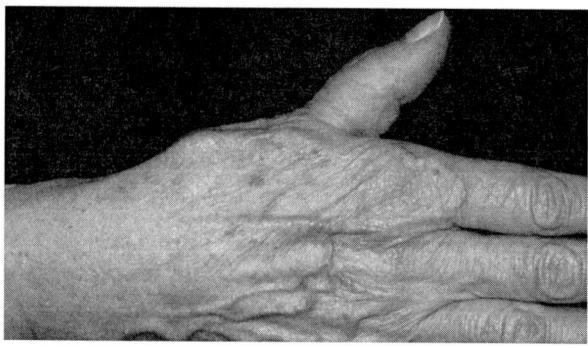

FIGURE 3.16 Osteoarthritis of the first CMC joint is frequently associated with squaring at the base of the thumb

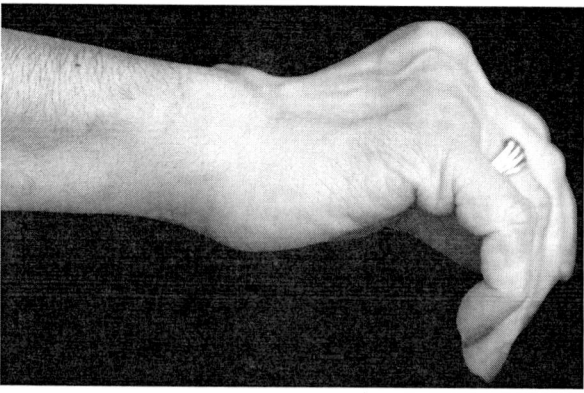

FIGURE 3.17 Palmar subluxation of the wrist in a patient with advanced rheumatoid arthritis

The wrist should flex about 80° and extend to approximately 70°. With the hand closed, the tips of the fingers should press hard into the palm of the hand (Fig. 3.18). Extension of the fingers should be smooth, with no "snatching," and reach 0° extension in all the joints (45–60°, in the thumb interphalangeal).

If mobility is at all limited, repeat the movements passively. There are two possibilities: (a) passive range of movement is no greater than active or (b) passive mobility is clearly wider than active.

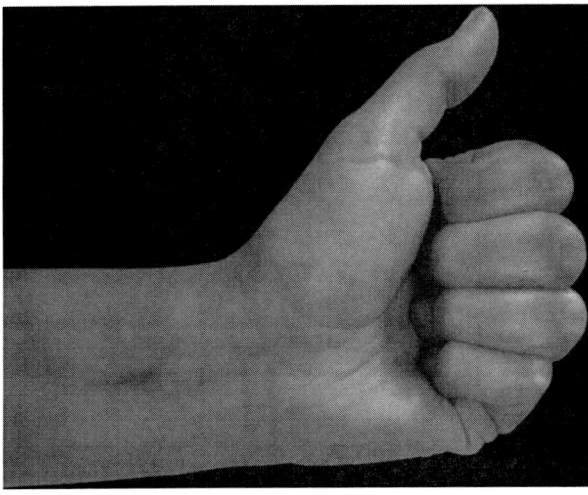

FIGURE 3.18 Active flexion of the fingers: fingertips should press firmly on the palmar aspect of the hand

What do these differences mean?

If the patient can carry out full active movements, we will be reassured that there is no major damage. Limitations in active as well as in passive movement indicate that the problem is structural, i.e. something is stopping the joints from moving completely: an articular lesion or fibrosis of the capsule. Passive mobility obviously does not require the patient's tendons, muscles, peripheral nerves or CNS. Lesions of these structures do not affect passive mobility, even if active movements are limited. Therefore, if passive mobility is more ample than active mobility, these structures should be assessed further.

The most common cause for this is tenosynovitis of the flexor tendons. In this very common condition, one or more fingers do not touch the palm of the hand, though we can make them do it easily. The presence of trigger movements of the finger suggests stenosing tenosynovitis.

In Dupuytren's contracture, the patient is unable to extend completely his ring finger (more rarely, the middle or little finger), due to hard thickening of the palmar fascia that holds the flexor tendons (Fig. 3.19).

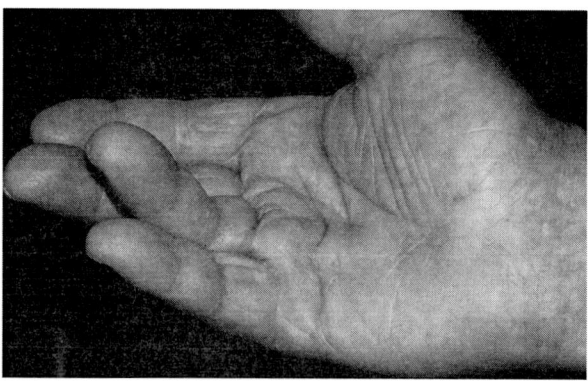

FIGURE 3.19 Dupuytren's contracture. Notice the thickening and contraction of the palmar fascia, proximal to the fourth finger. Active and passive extension of the fourth finger was limited

Palpation

a) Palpate any visible nodules
Feel their consistency, texture and location.

Rheumatoid nodes can affect the hands. They are firm, rubbery and painless and adhere to the deep fascial planes (Fig. 3.13a). The surface of gouty tophi (Fig. 3.13b) is irregular and sometimes whitish. They may deform slightly on pressure, with crepitus. Bouchard's and Heberden's nodes (on the proximal and distal interphalangeal joints, respectively, Fig. 3.14) are typical of nodal osteoarthritis of the hands. They have a bony consistency, (they comprise osteophytes) and are usually painless. Synovial cysts (ganglia), usually in the vicinity of the wrist, are soft and malleable.

Almost all of us have two small palpable nodes, one on either side of the palmar face of first metacarpophalangeal joint. What could they be?[2]

---

[2]Sesamoid bones.

b) Palpate the joints of the wrist

Use the back of your hand to check for local increase in temperature. Hold the patient's hand between yours and use your thumbs to explore the articular space between the radius and the carpus. Also palpate the processes of the radius and ulna on the lateral and medial face of the wrist, respectively (Fig. 3.20). If you find swelling on the back of the wrist, try to distinguish between tenosynovitis of the extensors and arthritis of the wrist, mobilizing the patient's fingers while palpating (in tenosynovitis, the swelling may move slightly with the mobilized tendon).

It is important to feel the bony contours under your fingers. The loss of typical definition indicates that there is something additional between your fingers and the bone – probably an inflamed synovium. The articular space of the radiocarpal joint is not easy to define as the edges of the articular surfaces are rounded and do not provide a clear, palpable reference. Experience acquired by repeating this assessment on all patients markedly increases the ability to detect small degrees of swelling. Pain on palpation along the articular space also suggests local inflammation.

c) Explore the possibility of de Quervain's tenosynovitis

The tendons affected in this condition form the anterior (palmar) border of the so-called anatomical snuffbox. If there is inflammation, palpation is painful. This pain may be exacerbated if the thumb is placed in resisted abduction (Fig. 3.21).

Finkelstein's maneuver is very sensitive and specific to this condition. Ask the patient to hold his thumb between the clenched fingers of his hand. Hold the patient's hand and firmly induce passive adduction (Fig. 3.22). Pain in the outer edge of the wrist is typical of de Quervain's tenosynovitis. Osteoarthritis of the 1st CMC joint can also cause pain on the lateral aspect of the wrist but not in Finkelstein's maneuver.

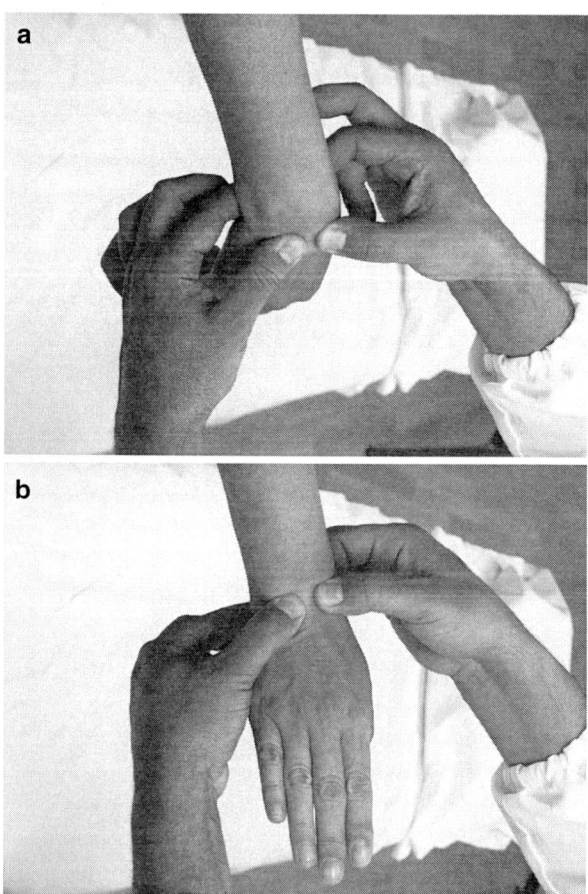

FIGURE 3.20 Palpation of the wrist. (**a**) and (**b**) The index fingers of the examiner palpate the palmar aspect of the wrist. The thumbs explore the joint line for tenderness, swelling or crepitus, while the wrist is passively flexed and extended. Palpate also the radial (**c**) and ulnar (**d**) processes

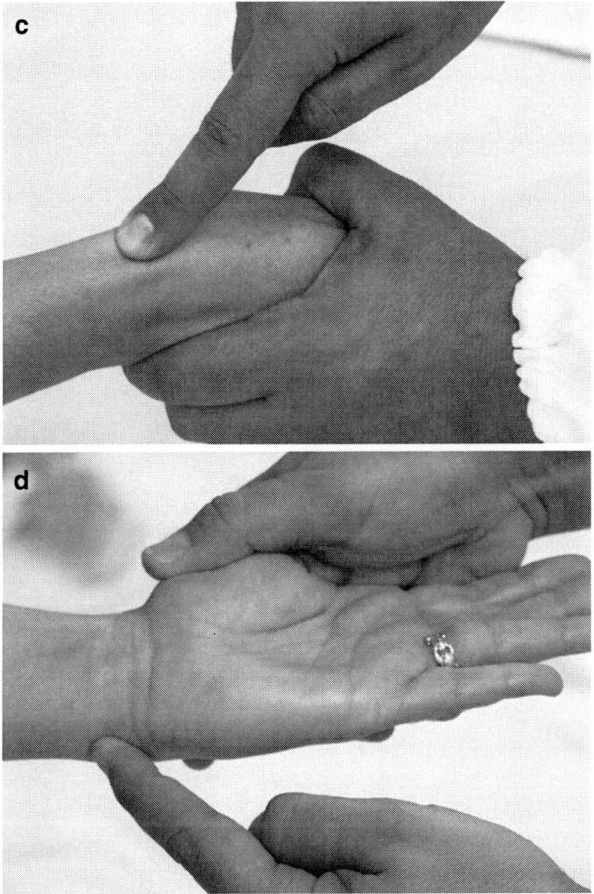

FIGURE 3.20 (continued)

d) Palpate the metacarpophalangeal joints (2nd to 5th)
The patient leaves his hand at rest. Place the MCPs at
about 45° flexion and insert your index finger behind these
joints and pull them gently towards you. Now palpate the
articular space and borders using the pads of the thumb
and index finger of your other hand together (Fig. 3.23).

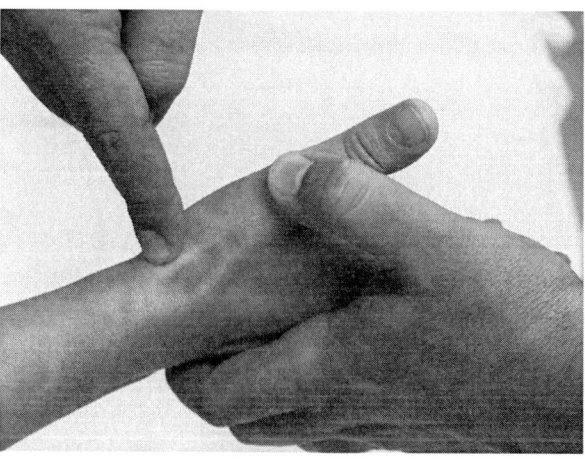

FIGURE 3.21 Palpation of the tendon sheath of the abductor pollicis longus and extensor pollicis brevis – De Quervain's tenosynovitis. Palpation during resisted abduction increases pain

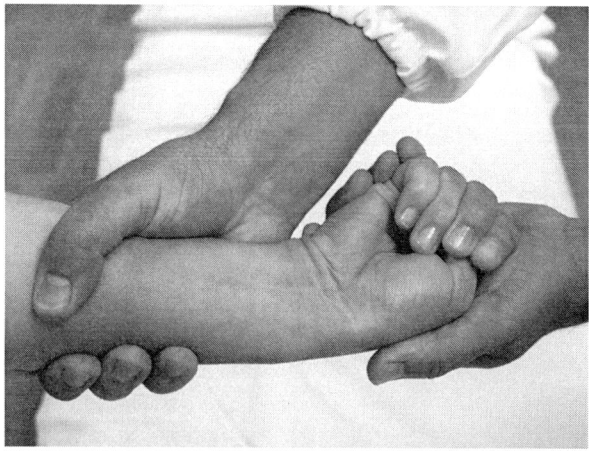

FIGURE 3.22 Finkelstein's maneuver. Positive in De Quervain's tenosynovitis

These spaces are clearly perceptible in normal hands. With experience, it is possible to identify even slight swelling of the synovium. The bony relief becomes ill-defined (increasing

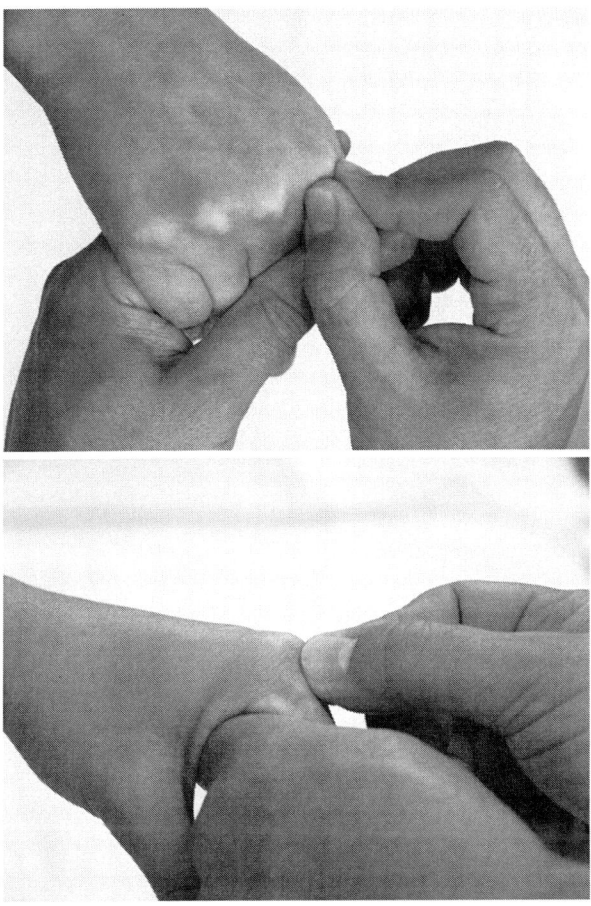

FIGURE 3.23 Palpation of metacarpo-phalangeal joints. The index finger of the examiner palpates the palmar aspect of the MCP while the sharpness of the joint line is explored with the tips of the index and thumb of the other hand

with higher degrees of inflammation). Note that the base of the first phalanx runs under the head of the metacarpal in flexion. The joint space is located 1.5–2 cm below the dorsal face of the metacarpal (Fig. 3.23b). An index finger placed under/behind the MCPs is very useful, as it makes the base of the phalanx more perceptible and pushes forward any articular effusion that there may be.

Repeat the operation for each joint of the four fingers (the MCP of the thumb is palpated differently). These joints are very often affected in rheumatoid arthritis, lupus, psoriatic arthritis, etc.

It is very rare to find bony (hard) swelling of the MCPs. This is typical of osteophytes and therefore osteoarthritis – which is unusual in this location.

> **e) Palpate the first MCP and the proximal interphalangeals**
>
> Place the pulps of your index finger and thumb on each side of the joint. They will act as sensors only, without moving. Place the thumb and index finger of your other hand on the dorsal and palmar faces of the joint, exerting and relieving pressure repeatedly (Fig. 3.24).

The synovium of these joints is strictly delimited by the capsule. If there is any swelling or articular effusion, the synovium acts like a small sac of water. When we palpate in an anteroposterior direction, there is transverse expansion that the sensor finger and thumb identify as fluctuation. The technique must be accurate to avoid mistakes.[3] Fluctuation suggests synovitis, i.e. arthritis. This interpretation is reinforced if palpation causes pain (there can be swelling without pain and pain without swelling).

These joints are often the site of inflammation in rheumatoid arthritis, psoriatic arthritis, lupus, etc.

---

[3]We all have fluctuation *between* the finger joints because the local soft tissue is enveloped by a fascia. Try to find fluctuation in someone else's phalanges. To avoid mistaking this sign for synovitis when assessing the interphalangeal joints, your fingers must only touch the patient's joint: use the tips of your fingers and not the whole of your distal phalange.

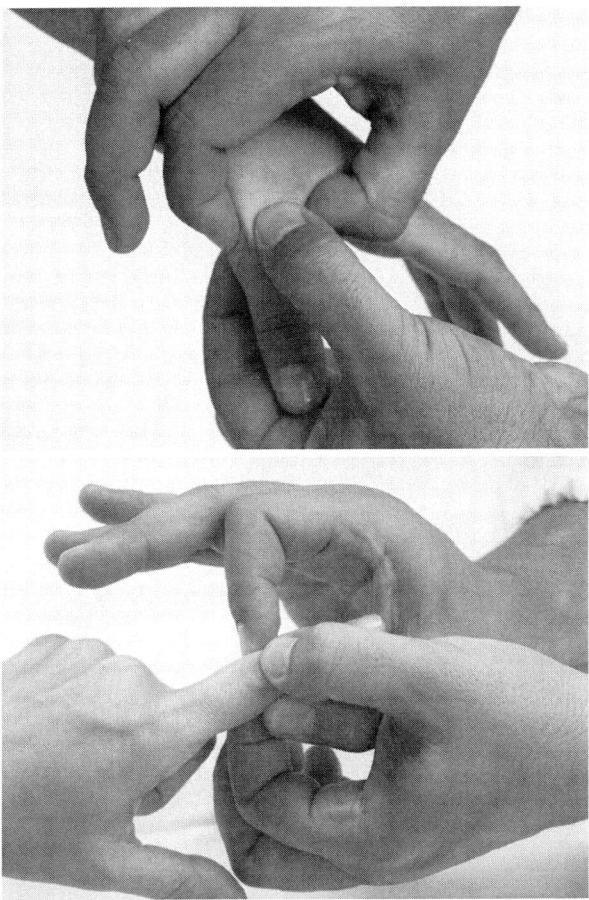

FIGURE 3.24 Palpation of the first metacarpo-phalangeal and proximal interphalangeal joints: look for tenderness and fluctuance

f) Palpate the distal interphalangeal joints

The method is similar to that used for the proximal interphalangeals (Fig. 3.25). Swelling is much rarer and fluctuation is not always perceptible because of the small volume of the

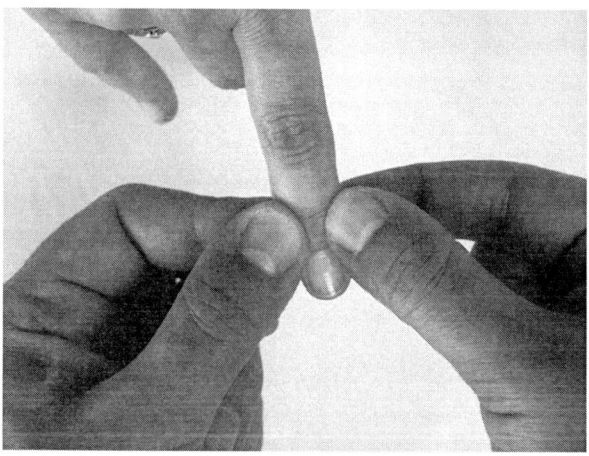

FIGURE 3.25 Palpation of the distal interphalangeal joints: look for tenderness, fluctuance and bony nodules

joint. The most common alteration here is Heberden's nodes (bony nodules that are typical of nodal osteoarthritis of the hands).

Inflammation of the DIPs is very suggestive of psoriatic arthritis, particularly when it is found in combination with nail pitting. Rheumatoid arthritis and lupus usually spare these joints.

g) Palpation of flexor tendons and their synovial sheaths
Place your thumb gently on the path of the flexor tendon of the index finger, on the palmar face of the hand, immediately above the metacarpophalangeal. Use it as a sensor while you passively flex and extend the patient's finger, holding it by the distal phalange (Fig. 3.26). Repeat the maneuver with the other fingers.

Assessment of the flexor tendons is especially important if there is limitation of active flexion of the fingers but not of

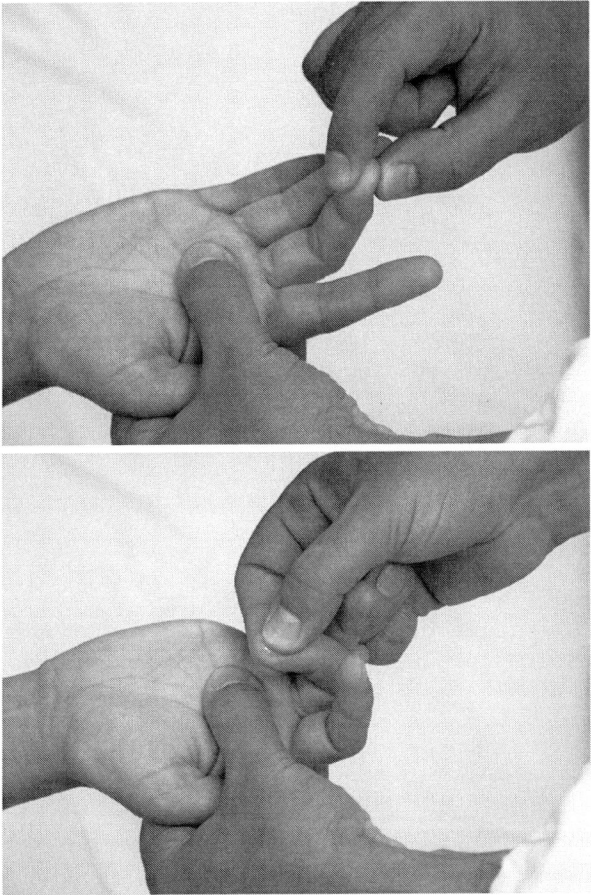

FIGURE 3.26 Palpation of flexor tendon sheaths. The thumb feels for crepitus, swelling or nodules adherent to the tendon, while the finger is passively mobilized

passive mobilization. In tenosynovitis you will feel thickened tissue gliding under the palpating fingers, sometimes with crepitus and pain. This is an inflamed synovial sheath, which is dragged by the tendon to which it adheres. In the case of trigger finger, look for a nodule adhering to and moving with the tendon, which is almost always perceptible.[4]

> **Note**
> The distribution of the affected joints in the wrist and hand and the types of changes are very important for differential diagnosis of the most common joint diseases in this area (Fig. 3.27).
>
> The accompanying alterations – manifestations on the skin or nails, nodules, malalignment, etc. – also help the diagnosis.

The Neurological Examination

A neurological examination is particularly indicated if the prior assessment suggests neurogenic pain: paresthetic pain, predominating at night, suggestive location, related to movements of the neck, weakness, etc.

Atrophy of the thenar and hypothenar eminences on the palmar face of the hand is also suggestive.

> **h) Assessing muscle strength**
> Successively test the patient's strength in the following movements (Fig. 3.28):
> - Extension of the wrist (root C7, radial nerve)
> - Opposition of thumb and index finger (root C7/8, median nerve)
> - Resisted flexion of the fingers (root C6–C8, median nerve)
> - Spreading the fingers (root C8/T1, ulnar nerve)

---

[4] The nodule that we feel is a thickening of the tendon itself, located near the opening of the tendon sheath. When the patient flexes his fingers hard, the nodule is forced into the sheath. When extending them again, he has to make an effort for the nodule to overcome the resistance of the entrance to the sheath. This forced exit results in a trigger movement, though once it is out it moves freely.

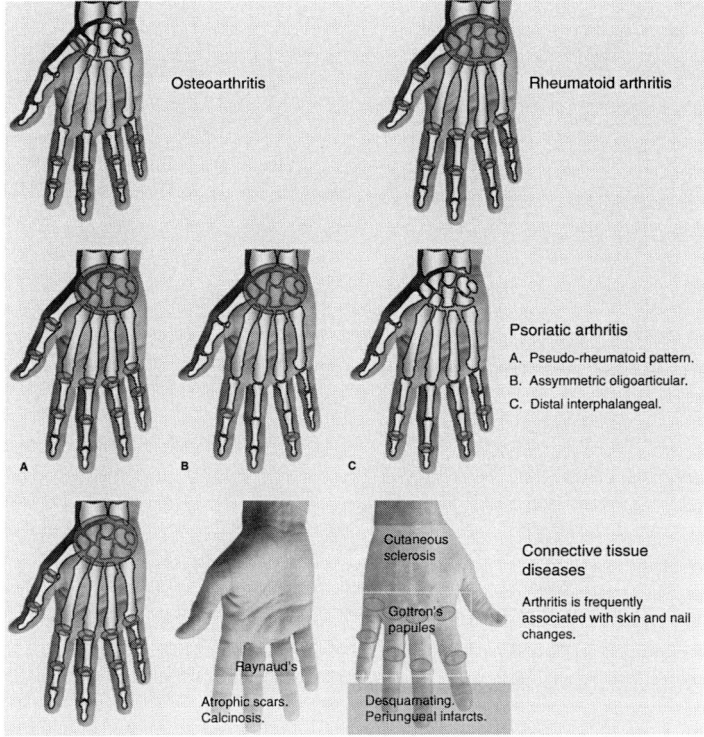

FIGURE 3.27 Writs and hand joints typically involved in the different arthropathies

i) Assessing sensitivity to pain

Hypoesthesia of the hand is only found in very advanced root or nerve lesions and is not necessary to prove a neurogenic lesion. Its assessment should take into account the sensory areas of the peripheral nerves (Fig. 3.4) and the radicular dermatomes.

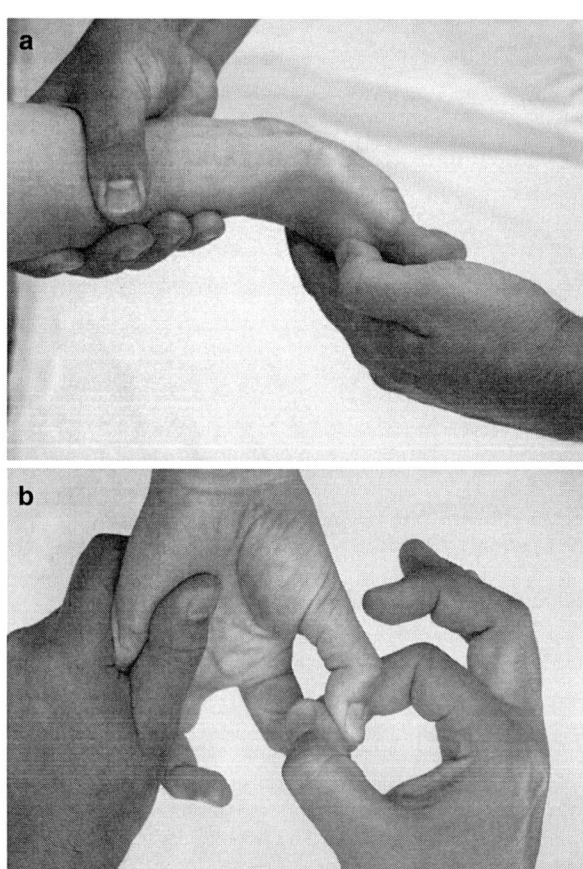

FIGURE 3.28 Neurological examination of the hand and wrist. (**a**) Extension of the wrist (C7, radial nerve). (**b**) Opposition of the thumb and index finger (C7–C8, median nerve). (**c**) Resisted flexion of the fingers (C6–C8, median nerve). (**d**) Spreading of the fingers (C8-T1, ulnar nerve)

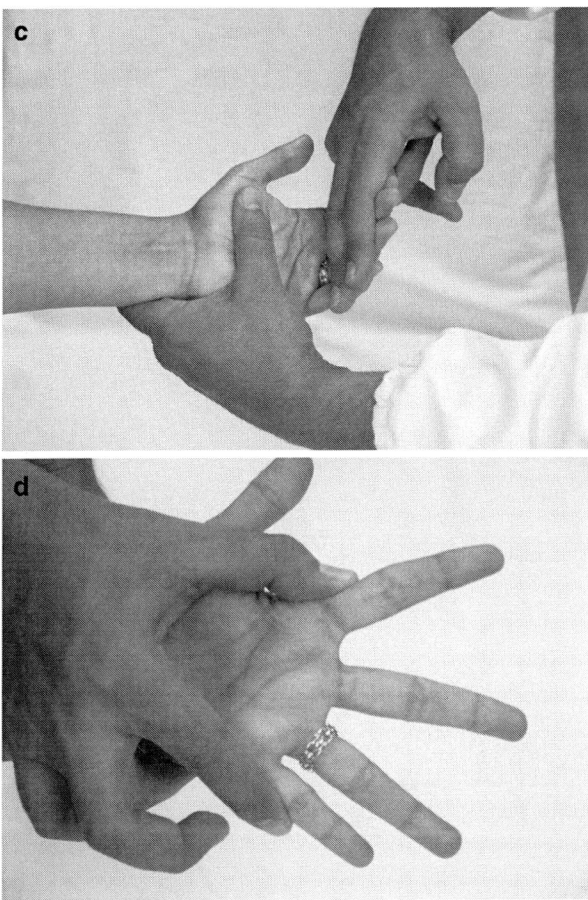

FIGURE 3.28 (continued)

j) Tinel's sign

Tinel's sign is checked by percussion on a point of the path of a nerve. It is positive if it results in dysesthesia radiating to the sensory area of the nerve (it sometimes radiates

proximally). Depending on the area affected by the spontaneous "neurogenic" symptoms, you may perform:
- Tinel of the median nerve in the carpal tunnel (Fig. 3.29a);
- Tinel of the ulnar nerve in Guyon's canal (Fig. 3.29b);
- Tinel of the ulnar nerve in the elbow (Fig. 3.30c).

k) Phalen's test
Place the patient's wrists in forced flexion so that the backs of his hands press against each other for about 60 seconds (Fig. 3.30). In carpal tunnel syndrome this test often reproduces symptoms: paresthesia in the territory of the median nerve.

Typical Cases
3.A. Pain in The Hands (I)
Maria de Jesus, a 54-year old cook, said that she was finding it increasingly difficult to do her job. She would wake up several times a night with pain in her hands, especially her right one, which prevented her from sleeping. The pain was relieved by moving her hands. She felt that her hands were "swollen" and "numb" in the morning. This usually got better with time, but she was "clumsy." She kept dropping things (she had broken more dishes in the last 3 months than in the rest of her life!). She denied pain in any other locations, except for the mechanical back pain that she had been having for about 10 years. During our systematic enquiry she said that she had been feeling tired and forgetful but that it was "probably lack of sleep." She had recently put on 6 kg.

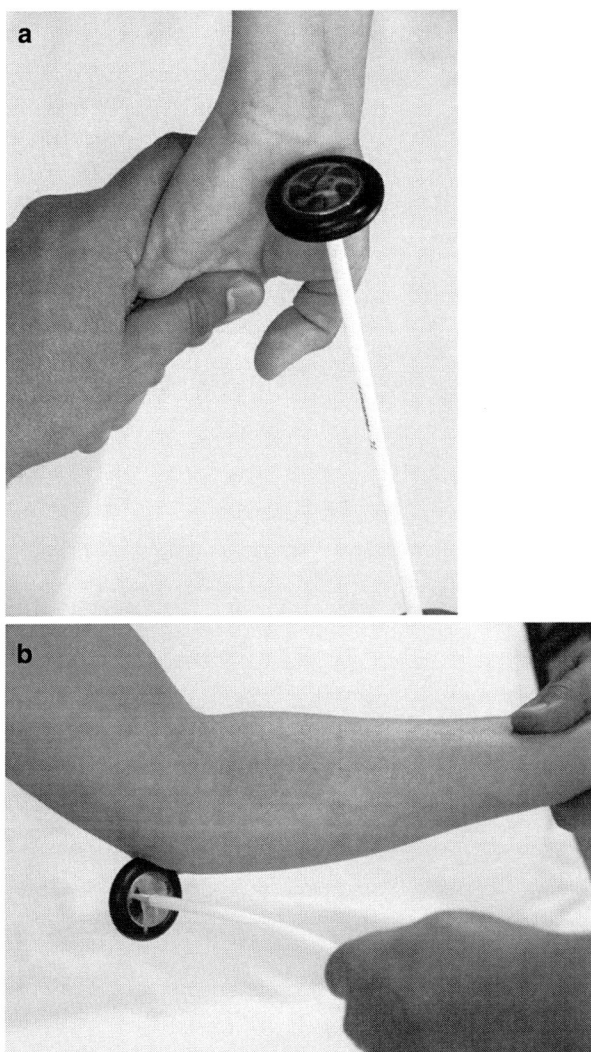

FIGURE 3.29 Tinel's sign. (**a**) Tinel of the median nerve in the carpal tunnel. (**b**) Tinel of ulnar nerve in the ulnar tunnel. (**c**) Tinel of the ulnar nerve in the elbow

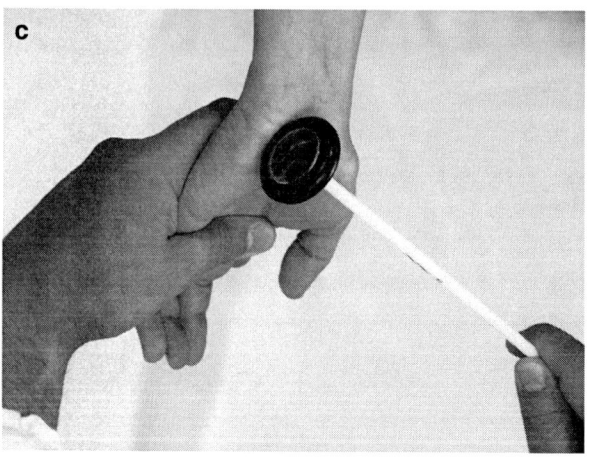

FIGURE 3.29 (continued)

Imagine the essential steps of the clinical examination that you would give her.

Our clinical examination revealed an obese patient (weight: 78 kg; height: 1.54 m) with no physical anomalies in the physical examination other than firm edema in her legs. The whole rheumatologic examination was normal, with no pain or limitation of movements. Her hands were also normal, with no swelling, muscular atrophy or alterations in the skin or nails. There were no limitations to active or passive mobility, and palpation was painless, with no signs of synovitis or tenosynovitis.

How would you explain her symptoms?
Would you conduct any further clinical assessments?

We asked the patient again about the pain. Yes, she had had some tingling. She said that her whole hand was affected but, when pushed, admitted that the little finger was not involved.

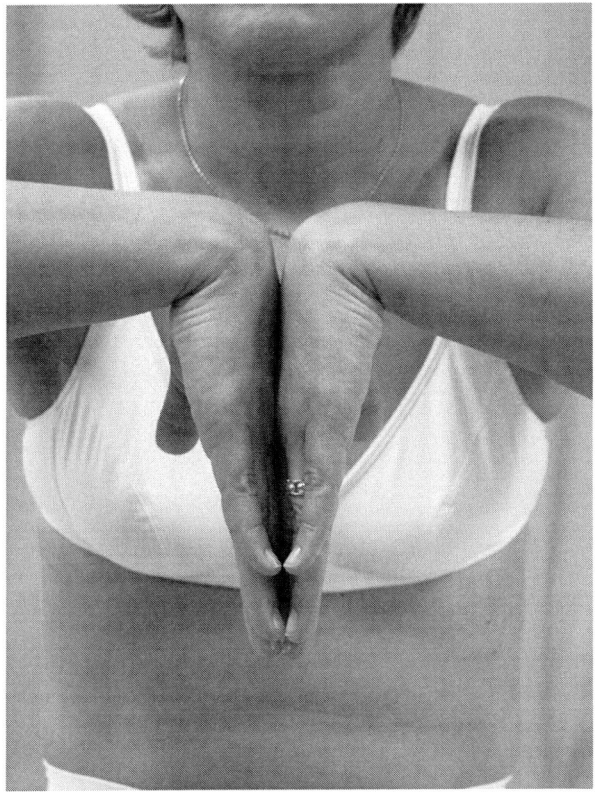

FIGURE 3.30 Phalen's test. This position is kept for about 1 minute: paresthesia in the median nerve distribution suggests carpal tunnel syndrome

We tested for Tinel's sign in the median nerve and conducted Phalen's test, both of which were positive bilaterally. The examination of the cervical spine was normal.

What are the possible diagnoses?
Would you request any diagnostic tests?
We confirmed the diagnosis of carpal tunnel syndrome, without additional tests.

Could the history of weight gain, edema and tiredness have some other significance?

We advised Maria de Jesus to wear a splint on her wrist and we asked for a thyroid hormone test. Two weeks later, the results confirmed the diagnosis of hypothyroidism, and she was started on thyroxin. We discussed alternative treatments with the patient and decided to postpone a possible corticosteroid injection into the carpal tunnel until after a course of thyroid replacement.

After 6 weeks, Maria de Jesus was "a new woman...".

Carpal Tunnel Syndrome
Main Points

This is a very common condition, especially in middle-aged women.

The main symptoms are pain and paresthesia of the median nerve area (or the whole hand...), mainly at night and in the morning, which improve with movement.

Patients often lose manual dexterity and describe diffuse, discreet swelling of the hands in the morning.

Clinical examination finds no signs of joint disease or limitation of movement.

Positive Tinel's and Phalen's tests reinforce the diagnosis.

Atrophy of the thenar eminence and loss of sensitivity in the median nerve territory are later manifestations.

Most cases have no identifiable underlying cause. Diabetes, hypothyroidism, pregnancy, work with vibrating machinery and intensive use of the hands are risk factors. It often accompanies synovitis or tenosynovitis of the wrist (e.g. in rheumatoid arthritis).

An electromyogram is justified in doubtful cases or if surgery is considered. Lab tests are only justified to look for the underlying cause and are oriented by clues collected in the general enquiry and examination.

Therapy consists basically of local protection (splints) and treatment of any identifiable underlying disease.

Corticosteroid injections can be administered in cases of intense or persistent symptoms. Decompression surgery is sometimes indispensable.

Typical Cases
3.B. Pain in The Hands (II)

It all seemed to have started at the age of 50, after the menopause. The patient had aches and pains here and there that she considered normal for her age. At the age of 56, the pain in her hands became persistent and daily. It was this pain that brought her to us at the age of 62. The pain appeared mainly after prolonged use of the hands (e.g. after crocheting for a long time, one of her favorite occupations that she could no longer do...). She often woke up with pain and stiffness in her hands lasting up to about an hour in the worst phases. She had only noticed swelling once, two years previously. The second DIP of her right hand had been swollen and red with a blister that had burst and produced some fluid. She had noticed progressive deformation in several joints. But, "Doctor, this must run in the family. My mother's hands were all deformed when she died. That's what worries me most..."

We asked her to show us her hands (Fig. 3.31) and point to exactly where it hurt. She indicated the base of her thumbs and, diffusely, the proximal and distal interphalangeal joints. The metacarpophalangeal joints and wrists were not affected. She also had typical mechanical pain in her knees and lumbar region.

Palpation of the trapeziometacarpal joints was painful.[5] Palpation of the PIPs and DIPs was painless, but there were firm nodules located on either side of the dorsal face of several joints. Finkelstein's maneuver was negative.

Give a brief description of this case.[6]

What is your diagnosis? Are there any alternative possibilities?

Would you ask for any diagnostic tests?

Would you like to consider the treatment?

Our clinical examination left no doubt. The patient had nodal osteoarthritis of the hands and osteoarthritis of the 1st carpo-metacarpal joints.

We explained the nature of the condition to the patient and told her that, unfortunately, there was no way of stopping its progression to deformity. We stressed, however, that patients with nodal osteoarthritis maintain good mobility and function in spite of the deformities. We suggested local application of heat and topical anti-inflammatory creams. We recommended paracetamol to relieve the pain when necessary, reserving anti-inflammatories for use if this measure failed.

---

[5] The 1st CMC (Trapeziometacrpal joint) can be palpated at the base of the thumb in the anatomical snuff box. The joint space is not perceptible but in osteoarthritis there is pain and osteophytes are occasionally perceptible.

[6] A 62-year old woman with mixed-rhythm pain in the small joints of her hands and progressive deformation with stony nodes.

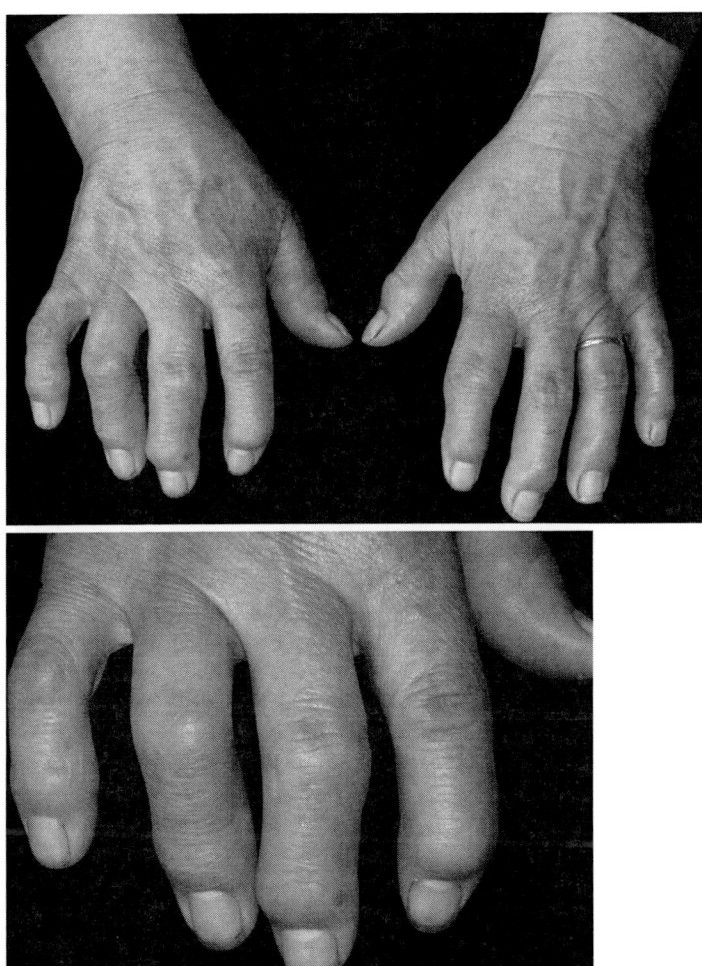

FIGURE 3.31 Clinical case "Pain in the hands (II)". Notice the nodular deformities around the PIPs and DIPs, as well as the deviations of some phalanges

Typical Cases
3.C. Pain in the Wrist (I)
Graça Oliveira, a 42-year old domestic employee, described increasingly intense pain in her left wrist and the distal part of her left forearm for about three weeks (she was left-handed). The pain worsened while she was working and continued to bother her somewhat even when at rest. There was no pain at night and no paresthesia. She denied any recent trauma and had noticed no signs of inflammation.

She had always been healthy and this was the first episode of such symptoms.

On examination, inspection and mobility of wrists and hands were normal. Palpation of the joints revealed no abnormalities, thus excluding the possibility of synovitis. Tinel's and Phalen's tests were negative.

Find out for yourself. What else is there to explain her pain?…

What aspects of the clinical examination haven't we explored?

That's right. Palpation of the tendons on the outer border of the wrist caused pain, which was more marked at the anterior edge of the anatomical snuffbox. We noted slight thickening in this tendon. Abduction or resisted flexion of the thumb caused pain similar to the spontaneous pain, exacerbated by simultaneous palpation of the tendon. Finkelstein's maneuver caused intense pain.

This allowed the diagnosis of De Quervain's tenosynovitis, without the need for additional diagnostic tests. We advised her to rest her left arm for about a week and recommended local friction with an anti-inflammatory cream after applying heat for 5–10 minutes. The patient came back 2 weeks later as she had not improved.

We then administered a careful injection of corticosteroid into the tendon sheath and recommended complete rest of the arm for 2 days. With the patient, we explored the possibility of diminishing repeated use of the thumb with special splint. She said that this was incompatible with her work.

A couple of weeks later she told us on the phone that she no longer had any symptoms. The risk of recurrence is high, however.

De Quervain's Tenosynovitis
Main Points

This consists of the inflammation of the tendon sheath of the long abductor and short extensor of the thumb.

It appears particularly in middle-aged women and is associated with repetitive manual work.

The pain is predominantly mechanical and located in the radial edge of the wrist, with some proximal or distal radiation.

The diagnosis is based on pain on local palpation, resisted mobilization and Finkelstein's maneuver.

The initial treatment involves rest and topical anti-inflammatories.

Local corticosteroid injection may solve the problem, but it must be carefully administered.[7]

Protecting the joint, with the use of appropriate splints is helpful in preventing recurrence.

---

[7]Injection of corticosteroids into the tendon weakens it and may lead to a subsequent rupture.

Typical Cases
3.D. Pain in the Hands (III)
The symptoms had been going on for about 4 months when we saw the patient for the first time. She described pain and inflexibility in both hands, especially in the morning. The stiffness sometimes lasted up to 2 hours. By the afternoon she had practically no symptoms. Her family doctor had prescribed anti-inflammatories, which relieved the pain without eliminating it all together. She attributed epigastric pain to this medication.

She denied any other articular or extra-articular complaints during a thorough enquiry.

The general clinical examination showed no alterations other than reduced active flexion of the fingers. Careful palpation of the metacarpophalangeal and interphalangeal joints was painless with no signs of articular swelling.

How would you continue investigating this case?

We tested passive mobility. It was quite easy to flex the fingers completely, much beyond active mobility. Palpation over the flexor tendons of the fingers, with simultaneous passive mobilization, was painful and showed clear thickening of the tissue adjacent to the flexor tendons of the index and middle fingers on the left and the index, middle and ring fingers on the right. There was discreet crepitus.

Arthritis of the Wrist and Hands
Main Points
Practically all types of arthritis can involve the hands.

The diagnosis of arthritis requires demonstration of joint inflammation, i.e. synovial swelling, on clinical examination.

The clinical examination technique should be thorough.

Monoarthritis of the wrists and hands is relatively rare. After excluding septic or microcrystalline arthritis, we should consider the possibility of incipient polyarthropathy.

The systematic enquiry and general examination are essential to the differential diagnosis.

The distribution of the affected joints in the wrists and hands is highly suggestive of the type of arthritis (Fig. 3.27).

The lab tests and treatment indicated depend on the overall clinical context.

Tenosynovitis often accompanies arthritis of the hands, and can be the first sign of this condition.

A diagnosis of inflammatory arthritis of any kind justifies sending the patient to a specialist as soon as possible.

What is your diagnosis?
Are any diagnostic tests necessary?
How would you interpret them?
What approach would you take?

Our examination showed that the patient had **tenosynovitis of the finger flexors**.

This condition in a young woman (aged 38), who did not do hard manual work and had no other manifestations, strongly suggested incipient polyarthritis.

We therefore changed her anti-inflammatory treatment, opting for a long-acting agent to be taken at night in order to guarantee maximum efficacy in the morning, associated with some gastric protection. We requested several lab tests: full blood count, sedimentation rate in the first hour, liver enzymes, creatinine, glucose, urinalysis, rheumatoid factor and antinuclear antibodies.

For personal reasons, the patient was only able to see us again 3 months later. The pain had become worse and so had

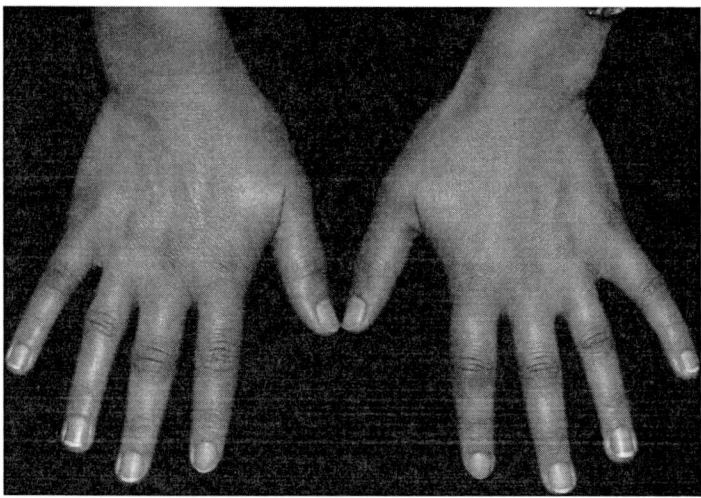

FIGURE 3.32 Clinical case "Pain in the hands (III)". Please note that although inspection suggests joint swelling, this can only be proved by palpation

the stiffness, which now lasted the whole morning. The pain kept her awake at night and now involved her right wrist and her toes. She had noticed edema in her hands about 2 months before (Fig. 3.32). She continued to deny any extra-articular manifestations of any kind. The epigastric pain had disappeared.

On examining her we now noticed a moderate reduction in flexion of the fingers, which could not be reduced passively. The signs of tenosynovitis persisted but were now accompanied by clear swelling, without redness, of the first, second and third MCPs on the left and the first and second on the right. There was fluctuation and pain on palpation of the right and left first, second and third PIPs and the third left PIP. Her right wrist was painful on palpation, with appreciable swelling and slight local heat. Transverse palpation of the metatarsal-phalangeal caused pain.

Give a brief description of this clinical condition.
What is your interpretation now?

There was now evidence of polyarthritis (inflammatory pain, with signs of inflammation in several joints), which was additive (as more joints were becoming involved), symmetrical (MCPs on each side, PIPs on each side) and predominantly peripheral (wrists and small joints of the hands), with no systemic manifestations. These characteristics are highly suggestive of rheumatoid arthritis. Psoriatic arthritis or another disease of the connective tissue was possible, even with no extra-articular manifestations.

When the lab tests came back, the blood count, creatinine and liver enzymes were normal. The sedimentation rate was high at 53 mm in the first hour. The rheumatoid factor and antinuclear antibodies were negative.[8]

We explained the situation to the patient and started her on appropriate treatment for rheumatoid arthritis.

Typical Cases
3.E. Pain in the Hands (IV)
Alice, aged 32, was referred to us by her GP because of pain in her hands, which had been developing for several months and was "unresponsive to non-steroidal drugs." The pain mainly affected the small joints of her hands, particularly at night and in the morning, with morning stiffness lasting from 30 to 60 minutes. She described mild hand swelling, particularly in the morning.

The pain was not incapacitating, but was still troublesome and worrying. She described transient episodes of intense pain in which her hands turned purple. These episodes were especially triggered by cold and emotional stress. No other joints were involved.

---

[8]NB: rheumatoid factor is only positive in about 75 % of cases of rheumatoid arthritis and this percentage is lower in the first months of the disease. The diagnosis is based on the clinical assessment even with a negative rheumatoid factor.

What possible diagnoses are you thinking of?
What additional information would you want?

The systematic enquiry was particularly interesting. The episodes of acute pain were accompanied by a clear change in color of some fingers (especially the index and middle finger of each hand), which first went very pale and later cyanotic. This had been happening for several years, particularly in winter, but she had never thought much of it. When asked, she said that she often had long-lasting painful mouth ulcers but denied any vaginal ulcers. Her eyes were frequently itchy and red, especially in the evening. Her skin had become quite sensitive to the sun the previous summer and she had suffered an erythematous reaction on her face and hands, which had gone away after a few weeks.

Her medical history included hospitalization due to pleural effusion with fever. This was attributed to pulmonary tuberculosis and had responded to treatment. All these "little things" had begun 4 years previously during her first pregnancy and she had been perfectly healthy until then.

Our general examination did not reveal any changes in her skin or mucosae. The chest examination was normal. Inspection of the hands found slightly spindle-shaped PIPs which were painful on palpation, but with no clear synovitis. There were small, scaly erythematous lesions on the backs of her fingers. Tinel's and Phalen's tests were negative.

The Hands in Connective Tissue Diseases
Main Points
All connective tissue diseases (CTDs) can cause joint pain or arthritis of the hands, which is often the first manifestation.

As a rule, synovitis is much more pronounced in rheumatoid arthritis than in other CTDs. There are often alterations of the skin and mucosae.

Always pay attention to inflammatory joint pain, especially in young people with no generalized pain.

A systematic enquiry and examination, focusing on the common extra-articular manifestations of CTDs, are the key to diagnosis.

Pay attention to the clinical information, even if none of it is conclusive, and consider the degree of probability of a systemic disease.

A clinically founded suspicion of CTD warrants requesting appropriate diagnostic tests and sending the patient to a specialist as soon as possible.

Briefly summarize this patient's problems.

- Peripheral, inflammatory polyarthralgia;
- Photosensitivity;
- Raynaud's phenomenon;
- Recurring mouth ulcers;
- Itchy eyes (xerophthalmia?);
- A history of pleurisy (tuberculosis?).

And all this in a young woman who we would expect to be healthy!

Review your possible diagnoses...

It's just as you think. We have sufficient information to suspect a systemic disease of the connective tissue. Note that, in practice, the difficulty of such cases lies in actively searching for and assessing relevant clinical data, which requires a systematic, focused enquiry and examination.

What diagnostic tests do you think are important?

The full blood count that we requested showed leucopenia, with normal red cell and platelet counts. Her liver enzymes and creatinine were normal. The urinalysis showed red cell castes with mild proteinuria and hematuria. Her sedimentation rate was high at 48 mm in the first hour, while reactive C protein was normal. Immunofluorescence for antinuclear antibodies was positive, at a titer of 1:320, with a homogeneous pattern.

The diagnosis of systemic lupus erythematosus was thus made. We set up some additional tests and prescribed the appropriate treatment.

Special Situations

Ulnar Nerve Syndrome

This is much less common than carpal tunnel syndrome. It causes paresthesia of the ulnar nerve territory, affecting only the medial border of the hand and fingers, if the compression is in Guyon's tunnel. The ulnar border of the forearm may also be involved if the compression is on the posteromedial aspect of the elbow joint. Positive Tinel's test at the sites of possible compression reinforces the diagnosis. There may be weakness in adduction of the little finger and hypoesthesia in the affected area. It requires differential diagnosis with C8 radiculopathy. An electromyogram may be necessary to confirm the diagnosis. Treatment involves avoiding local trauma by protecting the joints. If this is insufficient, it is worth administering a corticosteroid injection in the vicinity of the compression. Surgical decompression is necessary if the symptoms persist or if there are significant neurological signs.

Dupuytren's Contracture

This consists of fibrous thickening of the palmar fascia (i.e. not the tendons or tendon sheaths) thus preventing complete extension of the affected fingers, and leads to a fixed flexion deformity. The first and most commonly affected digit is the ring finger (Fig. 3.20). It is more common in men aged over 50. Palpation shows a hard, tense band. Diabetes mellitus, alcoholism and hard manual labor are predispositions, but most cases are idiopathic. There is a family predisposition.

Treatment is difficult and in the initial stages is aimed at protecting the area from repeated trauma and distending the tissues by means of local heat and extension exercises. Treatment of advanced, incapacitating forms usually requires surgery.

Trigger Finger

This is the result of stenosing tenosynovitis of the flexor tendon of one or more fingers. The patient describes pain in the palm while his finger often "gets stuck." In more advanced stages, the finger may remain fixed in flexion. It is released by active or passive extension of the finger, with pain and a triggering movement. Palpation of the flexor tendon and its sheath generally reveals a palpable node that moves with the tendon during passive mobilization. It can be improved by wearing splints and changes in the patient's daily activities. A corticosteroid injection may be highly effective. Surgery is occasionally needed.

Diabetic Hand Syndrome

A hands in diabetes are often the site of rheumatic complaints. Carpal tunnel syndrome, ulnar syndrome and tenosynovitis are the most common conditions in these patients.

Diabetic hand syndrome consists of a diffuse thickening of the soft tissues of the hand and fingers (fascia, tendons, capsules and ligaments), which limit mobility, particularly extension, without concomitant joint disease. It is known as diabetic chiroarthropathy and is usually painless. A typical feature of the clinical examination is the so-called **prayer sign**. Ask the patient to put his hands together as if praying. Patients with this condition find it difficult to join the palms of their hands due to the inability to extend completely the different joints (Fig. 3.33). The onset and progression of this syndrome occur in parallel with diabetic microangiopathy.

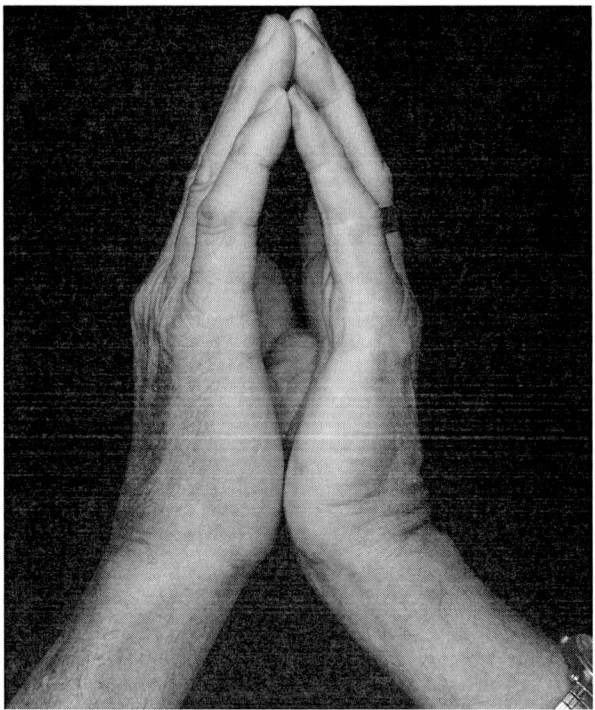

FIGURE 3.33 Prayer sign – diabetic chiroarthropathy (diabetic hand syndrome). The patient is unable to press both hands together

Treatment involves general care, physical therapy to maintain the elasticity of the tissues and tighter control of the diabetes.

Finger Clubbing: Hypertrophic Osteoarthropathy

Hypertrophic osteoarthropathy is a complex condition involving joint disease and generalized periostosis (periosteum inflammation and bone deposition). It usually appears in association with conditions such as lung diseases with chronic hypoxia, lung neoplasm, cyanotic heart disease, heavy smoking, liver cirrhosis, inflammatory gut disease, etc.

It is reflected by pain in a variety of locations. A burning sensation in the pads of the fingers is common. The lower limbs are often affected by deep, diffuse pain, which is typically worse when the legs are hanging.

Finger clubbing (or drumstick finger – Fig. 3.34) is one of its earliest, most common signs. The pads of the fingers thicken and swell and nails take on a convex shape. The perimeter of the finger at the base of the nail is larger than that of the DIP. Loss of space between the nails when we press two nail beds together is a particularly specific sign, reflecting loss of angle of nail bed (Fig. 3.34c).

Generalized Edema of the Hands

Occasionally a patient may describe generalized swelling of the hands, affecting not only the area around the joints but also the tissue of the back of the hand and wrist with pitting (boxer's hand).

This situation may rarely reflect acute or exacerbated arthritis, as in rheumatoid arthritis. The hand of a patient with scleroderma may suggest this condition as in its initial phases skin edema predominates before sclerosis.

Algodystrophy (or reflex sympathetic dystrophy) may cause diffuse edema of the hands with suggestive changes in color (mauve) and increased sweating.

The most common symptom of the rare condition RS3PE (remitting seronegative symmetric synovitis with pitting edema) is accentuated diffuse edema of both hands. It may respond perfectly to corticosteroid treatment but often progresses into typical rheumatoid arthritis.

Before considering these possibilities, however, do not forget to exclude other conditions like venous or lymphatic compression, allergic reaction or hypothyroidism.

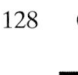

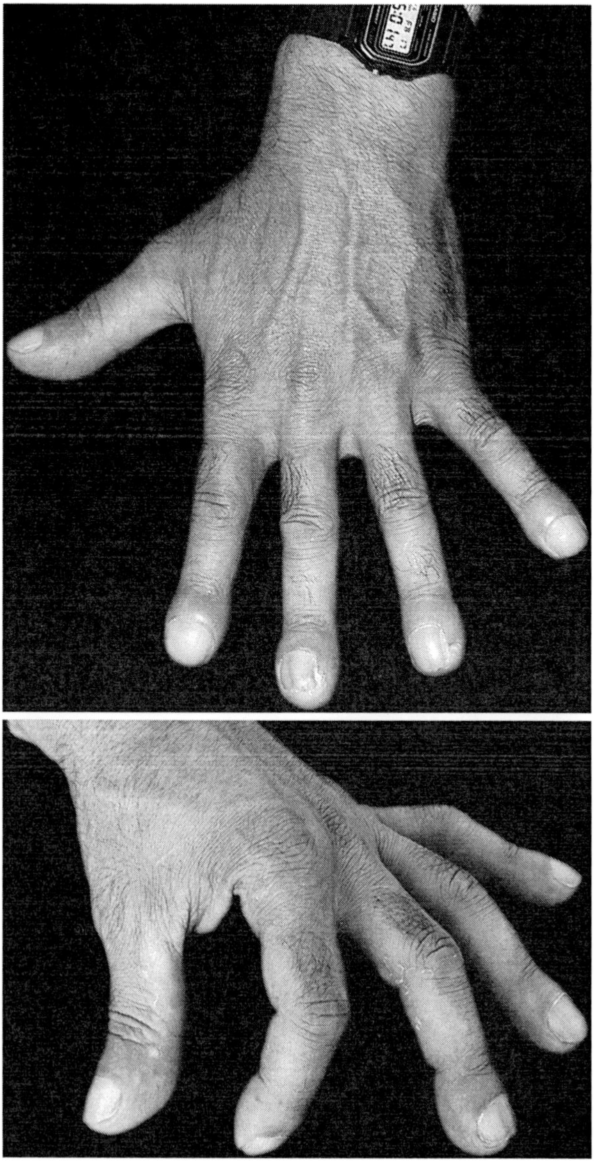

FIGURE 3.34 Clubbing. Notice the deformity of the distal phalanxes (clubbed fingers). Loss of the nailbed angle is an early sign of this condition

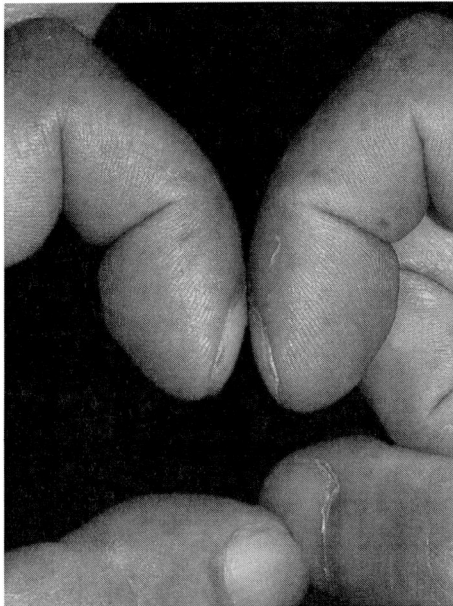

Figure 3.34 (continued)

Diagnostic Tests

A wide variety of rheumatic conditions of the wrist and hand may be diagnosed clinically, without the need for additional diagnostic tests. This is so for De Quervain's tenosynovitis, nodal osteoarthritis, osteoarthritis of the 1st CMC, Dupuytren's contracture, diabetic hand syndrome, and, to a large extent, rheumatoid arthritis, etc.

Carpal tunnel and ulnar tunnel syndrome do not normally require tests. An electromyogram may be justified if clinical assessment is not conclusive, if motor symptoms suggest severe median nerve compression and/or if surgery is likely. The need for tests to detect a pathology underlying these syndromes (glycemia, thyroid hormones, etc.) depends on the clinical context. As with many investigations, they are not very useful if requested indiscriminately.

If we suspect arthritis, there is a clear need for acute phase reactant studies, full blood count, basic biochemistry and other tests applicable to the diagnosis and to prepare for subsequent treatment. Rheumatoid factor and antinuclear antibodies are important tests in suspected polyarthritis, but they should never replace clinical assessment.

In rheumatology, no test can make the diagnosis in the absence of compatible clinical symptoms.[9]

Imaging

X-rays of the hands and wrists (anteroposterior and oblique angle) are justified whenever the clinical assessment suggests joint disease.

Reading these x-rays follows the same principles as for other joints:

Look at the alignment of the bones.
Assess the width and symmetry of the articular space.

Both arthritis and osteoarthritis involve loss of articular space. In arthritis, it tends to be homogeneous and uniform along the space. In osteoarthritis, the loss is often asymmetrical, depending on the lines of pressure exerted through the joint (Fig. 3.35).

Look at the bone density around the joints.

---

[9]A truth of La Palisse: for there to be rheumatoid arthritis, there must be… arthritis.

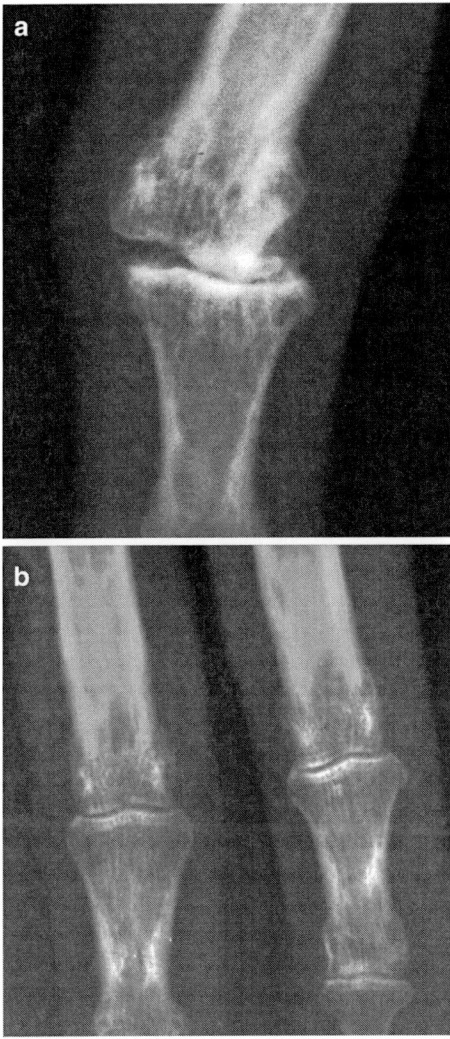

FIGURE 3.35 In osteoarthritis (**a**) joint space loss is usually focal or asymmetrical, while in inflammatory arthritis (**b**) it tends to be uniform and diffuse

When to Consider Arthritis of the Wrist and Hands
Main Points
Inflammatory pain
Rubbery swelling and/or pain in the joints on palpation
Signs of inflammation (inconstant)
Elevated acute phase reagents (usual)

In rheumatoid arthritis, periarticular osteopenia is one of its most typical signs and occurs early in the course of the disease. Conversely, osteoarthritis is associated with thickening of the subchondral bone – subchondral sclerosis. Curiously, although psoriatic arthritis is inflammatory, it does not cause pronounced osteopenia (Fig. 3.36).

Examine the edges of the joint for erosions or osteophytes.

Erosions look like small "bites" near the insertion points of the capsule and synovium. They are highly suggestive of rheumatoid arthritis and predominate in the joints usually affected by this type of arthritis: MCPs and PIPs. The styloid process of the ulna is also a common site of rheumatoid erosion. Lupus and other CTDs do not cause erosions, in spite of the articular inflammation.

In osteoarthritis, on the other hand, there are usually bony spurs (osteophytes) (Fig. 3.37).

Psoriatic arthritis is peculiar in this respect. It tends to cause erosions in the top of the proximal phalange and spurs in the base of the distal phalange, sometimes producing a "pencil in cup" appearance (Fig. 3.38).

Look for calcification of the cartilage or soft tissue – pay particular attention to the triangular ligament of the carpus (Fig. 3.39).

FIGURE 3.36 In rheumatoid arthritis (**a**) periarticular osteopenia is an early radiological feature. In osteoarthritis (**b**) subchondral bone sclerosis is a typical finding. Also notice the loss of joint space in both conditions

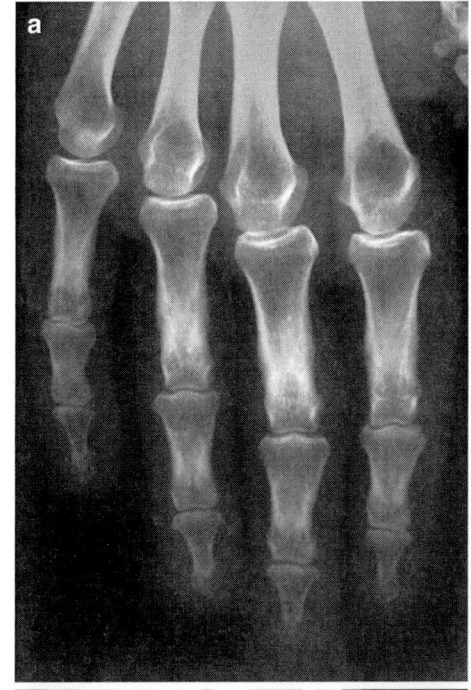

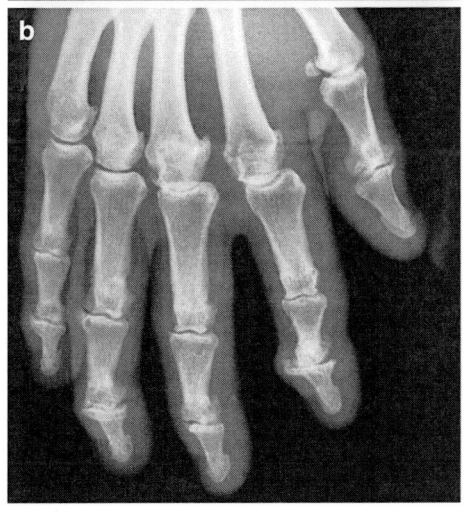

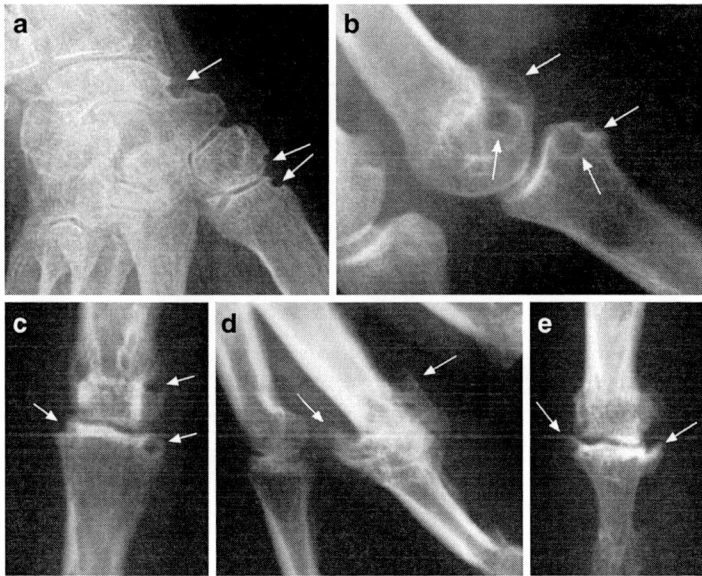

FIGURE 3.37 Erosions (focal areas of cortical bone resorption in the vicinity of joints) are common in rheumatoid arthritis (**a, b** and **c**). Conversely, in osteoarthritis bony projections at the joint margins, osteophytes, are typical (**d** and **e**)

Assess the distribution of the affected joints and compare it with the typical pattern of each joint disease.

Imaging of the Hands
Main Points
In simple terms, we can say that some radiological characteristics distinguish between the most common diseases of the wrist:
- Rheumatoid arthritis only removes bone (erosions and periarticular osteopenia)
- Osteoarthritis adds bone (osteophytes and subchondral sclerosis)
- Psoriatic arthritis does both (erosions and spurs, with no osteopenia or subchondral sclerosis) (Fig. 3.40)

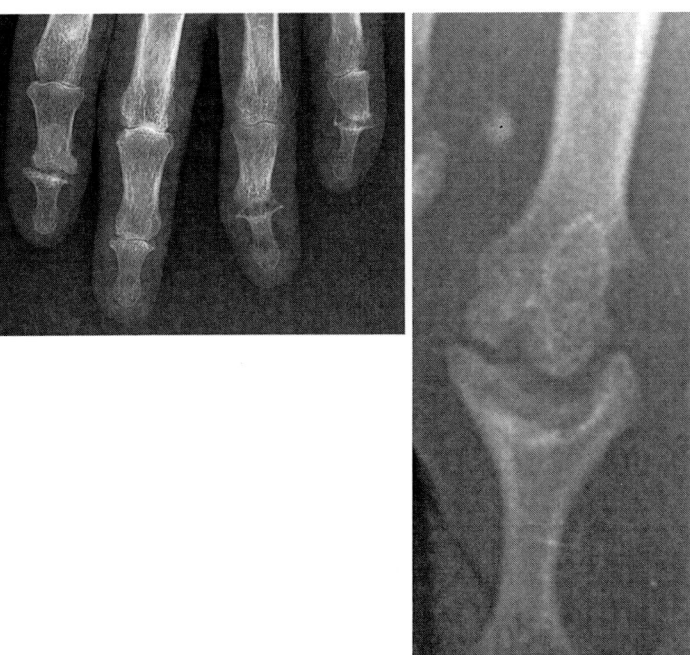

FIGURE 3.38 In advanced psoriatic arthritis, the association of erosions and exostoses may suggest so-called "pencil in cup" deformities

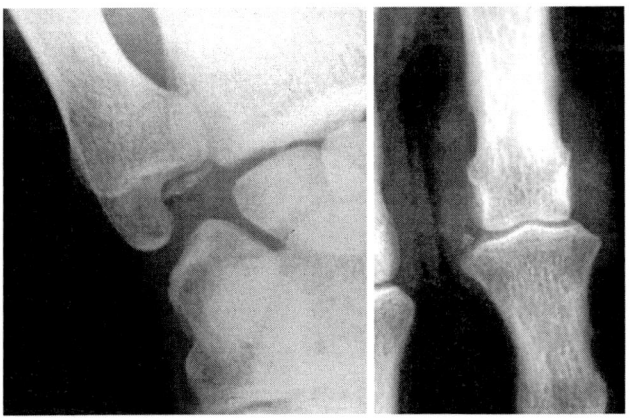

FIGURE 3.39 Chondrocalcinosis. Notice the calcification of the triangular ligament of the carpus and the interphalangeal joint

Bone scintigraphy is hardly ever justified to study the hands. Clinical assessment is highly informative and careful examination of the joints is usually more conclusive than scintigraphy.

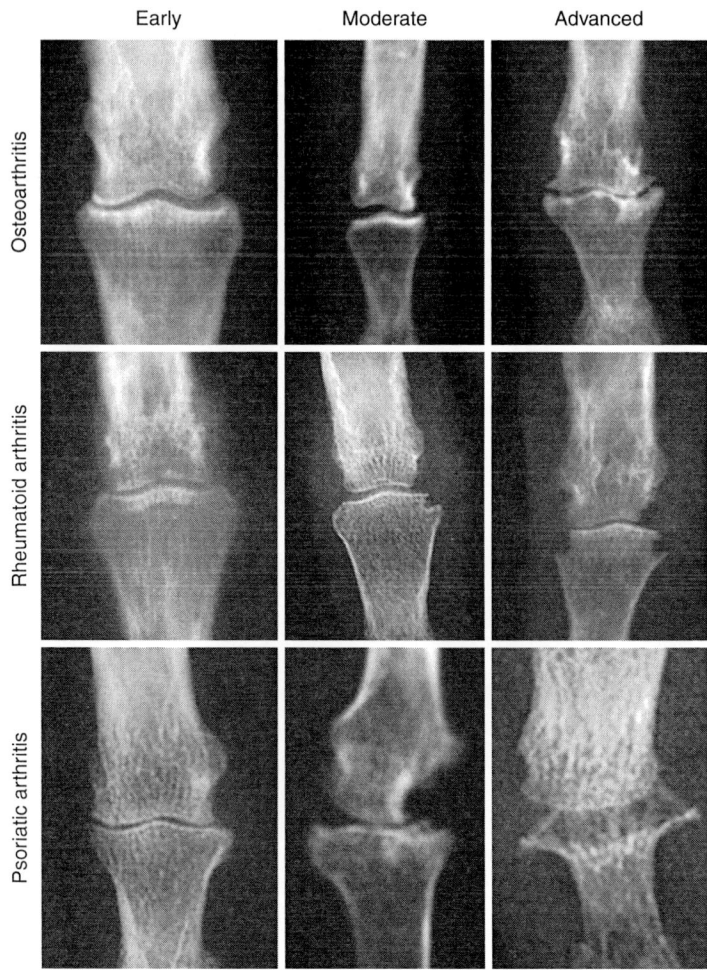

FIGURE 3.40 Typical radiological features of the three arthropathies in different stages of progression

Treatment

We have already dealt with the principles of treating lesions of the soft tissue and osteoarthritis of the hands. If pain and disability do not respond to medication, splints on the thumb or wrist can relieve the symptoms and improve mobility. Corticosteroid injections play an important part in treating some of these conditions, but should only be administered with a specific indication and by a trained physician.

When confronted with arthritis, a GP should refer the patient to a specialist as soon as possible. Even in chronic diseases like rheumatoid arthritis, the first few months are a crucial opportunity to avoid irreversible structural lesions, which is only possible with appropriate, timely treatment. Acute arthritis or suspected connective tissue disease warrant urgent referral.

If in doubt, GPs may request basic diagnostic tests such as acute phase reactants, rheumatoid factor or antinuclear antibodies, but should avoid wasting too much time using sophisticated tests, while awaiting an appointment with a consultant, you should resist the temptation to prescribe corticosteroids or immunosuppressants. Although they may provide rapid relief, it will be transient and there is a significant risk of side effects. Such hasty treatment may also blur the clinical features and influence results of diagnostic tests, making a definite diagnosis more difficult for the specialist. If you feel the need to resort to corticosteroids, consider whether your patient would not be better going to the ER at a hospital with a rheumatology department.

When Should the Patient be Referred to a Specialist?
Whenever and as soon as your clinical assessment demonstrates arthritis.

Whenever there are reasonable indications of connective tissue disease.

Whenever an x-ray shows loss of articular space or erosions, even if the clinical examination is not very suggestive.

Whenever soft tissue lesions are resistant to conservative treatment.

Index

J.A.P. da Silva, A.D. Woolf, *Rheumatology of the Upper
Limbs in Clinical Practice*, DOI 10.1007/978-1-4471-2242-5,
© Springer-Verlag London Limited 2012